Updates on Total Ankle Replacement

Editor

MARK E. EASLEY

FOOT AND ANKLE CLINICS

www.foot.theclinics.com

Consulting Editor
CESAR DE CESAR NETTO

March 2024 • Volume 29 • Number 1

ELSEVIER

1600 John F. Kennedy Boulevard • Suite 1800 • Philadelphia, Pennsylvania, 19103-2899

http://www.theclinics.com

FOOT AND ANKLE CLINICS Volume 29, Number 1
March 2024 ISSN 1083-7515, ISBN-978-0-443-18419-2

Editor: Megan Ashdown
Developmental Editor: Anita Chamoli

Foot and Ankle Clinics (ISSN 1083-7515) is published quarterly by Elsevier, Inc., 360 Park Avenue South, New York, NY 10010-1710. Months of issue are March, June, September, and December. Periodicals postage paid at New York, NY, and additional mailing offices. Subscription price per year is $369.00 (US individuals), $100.00 (US students), $397.00 (Canadian individuals), $100.00 (Canadian students), $514.00 (international individuals), and $215.00 (international students). For institutional access pricing please contact Customer Service via the contact information below. To receive student/resident rate, orders must be accompanied by name of affiliated institution, date of term, and the *signature* of program/residency coordinator on institution letterhead. Orders will be billed at individual rate until proof of status is received. Foreign air speed delivery is included in all *Clinics* subscription prices. All prices are subject to change without notice. **POSTMASTER:** Send address changes to *Foot and Ankle Clinics*, Elsevier Health Sciences Division, Subscription Customer Service, 3251 Riverport Lane, Maryland Heights, MO 63043. **Customer Service: 1-800-654-2452 (US and Canada). From outside of the United States and Canada, call 314-447-8871. Fax: 314-447-8029. E-mail: JournalsCustomerService-usa@elsevier.com (for print support); JournalsOnlineSupport-usa@elsevier.com (for online support).**

Reprints. For copies of 100 or more, of articles in this publication, please contact the Commercial Reprints Department, Elsevier Inc., 360 Park Avenue South, New York, NY 10010-1710. Tel.: 212-633-3874; Fax: 212-633-3820; E-mail: reprints@elsevier.com.

Printed in the United States of America.

Contributors

CONSULTING EDITOR

CESAR DE CESAR NETTO, MD, PhD
Orthopaedic Foot and Ankle Surgeon, Associate Professor, Department of Orthopedic Surgery, Duke University, Durham, North Carolina, USA

EDITOR

MARK E. EASLEY, MD
Duke Foot and Ankle Service, Duke University Health System, Durham, North Carolina, USA

AUTHORS

J. CHRIS COETZEE, MD
Twin Cities Orthopedics, Minneapolis, Minnesota, USA; Twin Cities Orthopedics, Eagan, Minnesota, USA

CONSTANTINE DEMETRACOPOULOS, MD
Associate Professor of Orthopaedic Surgery, Foot and Ankle Service, Hospital for Special Surgery, New York, New York, USA

SUNIL DHAR, MBBS, MS, MCh Orth, FRCS Ed Orth
Consultant Orthopaedic Surgeon, Foot and Ankle Unit, Nottingham Elective Orthopaedics, Nottingham University Hospitals City Campus, Nottingham, United Kingdom

M. PIERCE EBAUGH, DO
Attending Orthopedic Surgeon, Jewett Orthopedic Institute at Orlando Health, Winter Park, Florida, USA

PAULO N.F. FERRAO, MBChB (Pret), FCS Ortho (SA)
Surgeon, The Orthopaedic Foot and Ankle Unit, Netcare Linksfield Hospital; Consultant, Department of Orthopaedic Surgery, University of the Witwatersrand, Johannesburg, South Africa

AMANDA N. FLETCHER, MD, MS
Fellowship-Trained Foot and Ankle Orthopaedic Surgeon, OrthoCarolina Foot & Ankle Institute, Charlotte, North Carolina, USA

FRANCISCO FONTAN, MD
Resident, of Orthopaedics, University of Colorado School of Medicine, Aurora, Colorado, USA

KAMRAN HAMID, MD, MPH
Associate Professor, Department of Orthopaedic Surgery, Loyola University Medical Center, Maywood, Illinois, USA

DANIEL HAVERKAMP, MD, PhD
Orthopedic Surgeon, Department of Orthopedic Surgery, Xpert Clinics, SCORE Foundation, Specialized Center of Orthopedic Research and Education, Amsterdam, the Netherlands

KENNETH J. HUNT, MD
Associate Professor and Director, of Orthopaedics, University of Colorado School of Medicine, Aurora, Colorado, USA

JORIS P.S. HERMUS, MD
Orthopaedic Surgeon, Department of Orthopaedic Surgery, Research School CAPHRI, Maastricht University Medical Center +, Maastricht, the Netherlands

CRISTIAN INDINO, MD
Surgeon, Ortopedia della Caviglia e del Piede, Humanitas San Pio X, Milan, Italy

BAKUR A. JAMJOOM, BMBS, ChM, FRCS Orth, FRCS (T & O)
Leeds Teaching Hospitals, Chapel Allerton Hospital, Leeds, United Kingdom

JAEYOUNG KIM, MD
Research Fellow, Foot and Ankle Service, Hospital for Special Surgery, New York, New York, USA

VEIT KRENN, MD
Prof Dr med Dr med habil, Pathologie Trier, Trier, Germany

RYAN LEDUC, MD
Resident Physician, Department of Orthopaedic Surgery, Loyola University Medical Center, Maywood, Illinois, USA

CAMILLA MACCARIO, MD
Ortopedia della Caviglia e del Piede, Humanitas San Pio X, Milan, Italy

WILLIAM C. McGARVEY, MD
Fellowship Director, Orthopedic Foot and Ankle Reconstruction, McGovern College of Medicine, The University of Texas Health Science Center at Houston, Houston, Texas, USA

INMACULADA MORACIA-OCHAGAVIA, MD
Consultant Orthopedic Surgeon, Department of Orthopedic Surgery, La Paz University Hospital-IdiPaz, Madrid, Spain

JACO J. NAUDE, FC ORTHO (SA), MMed Orth (Pret)
Surgeon, The Orthopaedic Foot and Ankle Unit, Netcare Linksfield Hospital, Johannesburg, South Africa; Life Wilgers Hospital, Pretoria, South Africa

KATHRIN PFAHL, MD
Dr med, Department of Foot and Ankle Surgery, Schön Klinik München Harlaching—FIFA Medical Centre, Department of Orthopaedics and Trauma Surgery, Musculoskeletal University Center Munich (MUM), University Hospital, LMU Munich, Munich, Germany

EMERITO CARLOS RODRIGUEZ-MERCHAN, MD, PhD
Consultant Orthopedic Surgeon (Emeritus), Department of Orthopedic Surgery, La Paz University Hospital-IdiPaz, Madrid, Spain

DANIEL ROSS, MD
Orthopaedic Surgeon, Department of Orthopaedics, University of Colorado School of Medicine, Aurora, Colorado, USA

NIKIFOROS P. SARAGAS, FCS (SA) Ortho, PhD (Wits)
Department of Orthopaedic Surgery, University of the Witwatersrand; Orthopaedic Surgeon, The Orthopaedic Foot and Ankle Unit, Netcare Linksfield Hospital, Johannesburg, South Africa

CHRISTOPHER TRAYNOR, MD
Fellow, Twin Cities Orthopedics, Minneapolis, Minnesota, USA

FEDERICO G. USUELLI, MD
Ortopedia della Caviglia e del Piede, Humanitas San Pio X, Milan, Italy

LAURENS W. VAN DER PLAAT, MD
Orthopedic Surgeon, Department of Traumatology and Orthopedic Surgery, St.-Antonius-Hospital Kleve, Klinik für Unfallchirurgie und Orthopädie, Kleve, Germany

NIEK C. VAN DIJK, MD, PhD
Professor, Department of Orthopedic Surgery, University of Amsterdam, Amsterdam UMC location AMC, Amsterdam Zuidoost, the Netherlands; Head of Ankle Unit, FIFA Medical Centre of Excellence Ripoll-DePrado Sport Clinic, Madrid, Spain; Head of Ankle Unit, FIFA Medical Centre of Excellence Clínica do Dragão, Porto, Portugal; Casa di Cura San Rossore, Pisa, Italy

LAURIAN J.M. VAN ES, MD
Resident, Department of Orthopedic Surgery, Tergooi Clinics, Hilversum, the Netherlands; Xpert Clinics, SCORE Foundation, Specialized Center of Orthopedic Research and Education, Amsterdam, the Netherlands

MARKUS WALTHER, MD
Prof Dr med Dr med habil, Department of Foot and Ankle Surgery, Schön Klinik München Harlaching—FIFA Medical Centre, Department of Orthopaedics and Trauma Surgery, Musculoskeletal University Center Munich (MUM), University Hospital, LMU Munich, München, Germany; Department of Orthopedic Surgery, University of Wuerzburg, Würzburg, Germany; Paracelsus Medical University, Salzburg, Austria

DANIEL ROSS, MD
Orthopaedic Surgeon, Department of Orthopaedics, University of Colorado School of Medicine, Aurora, Colorado, USA

NIKIFOROS P. SARAGAS, FCS (SA) Ortho, PhD (Wits)
Department of Orthopaedic Surgery, University of the Witwatersrand; Orthopaedic Surgeon, The Orthopaedic Foot and Ankle Unit, Netcare Linksfield Hospital, Johannesburg, South Africa

CHRISTOPHER TRAYNOR, MD
Fellow, Twin Cities Orthopedics, Minnetonka, Minnesota, USA

FEDERICO G. USUELLI, MD
Ortopedia dello Sport e dell'Arto Inferiore, San Pio X, Milano, Italy

LAURENS W. VAN DER PLAAT, MD
Orthopedic Surgeon, Department of Traumatology and Orthopedic Surgery, St. Antonius Hospital, Klinik für Unfallchirurgie und Orthopädie, Kleve, Germany

NIEK C. VAN DIJK, MD, PhD
Emeritus, Department of Orthopedic Surgery, University of Amsterdam, Amsterdam UMC, location AMC, Amsterdam Zuidoost, The Netherlands; Head of Ankle Unit, FIFA Medical Centre of Excellence Ripoll-DePrado Sport Clinic, Madrid, Spain; Head of Ankle Unit, FIFA Medical Centre of Excellence Clinica do Dragão, Porto, Portugal; Casa di Cura San Rossore, Pisa, Italy

ZACHARIAH W. PINTER, MD
Resident, Department of Orthopaedic Surgery, Mayo Clinic, Minnesota, USA

MARKUS WALTHER, MD
Schön Klinik München Harlaching, Center for Foot and Ankle Surgery, Munich, Germany

Editorial Advisory Board

Contents

Preface: What You Will Find in this Collection of Current Total Ankle Arthroplasty Articles   xv

Mark E. Easley

Quality of Outcomes Research in Total Ankle Arthroplasty   1

Kamran Hamid and Ryan LeDuc

> Total ankle arthroplasty is a topic that has recently gained increasing inter-est, largely due to the improved outcomes, which have been demonstra-ted by short- and mid-term research studies on the newer, third-generation implant designs. The purpose of this review is to provide an up-dated assessment of the quality of outcomes research on total ankle arthroplasty.

Clinical Outcomes and Registry Data in Total Ankle Arthroplasty   11

Kenneth J. Hunt, Daniel Ross, and Francisco Fontan

> Total ankle arthroplasty (TAA) is an effective treatment for end-stage ankle arthritis consistently demonstrating good to excellent outcomes, even when considering factors such as deformity, patient age, bilaterality, and arthritis etiology. There is little consensus in the literature with regard to preferred patient-reported outcome metrics (PROMs) for assessing out-comes, although all metrics generally improve following TAA. Several countries have successful registries to track longevity of TAA in popula-tions; however, PROMs are generally not successfully tracked in registries. A trend toward consensus on outcome metrics and collaborative registries is warranted to optimize patient selection and outcomes in TAA

Results of Total Ankle Arthroplasty Versus Ankle Arthrodesis   27

Emerito Carlos Rodriguez-Merchan and Inmaculada Moracia-Ochagavia

> No differences have been found between total ankle arthroplasty (TAA) and ankle arthrodesis (AA) with respect to patient-reported outcome measures (PROMs), although both interventions were shown to improve PROMs with respect to the preoperative situation. That is, both interven-tions (AA and TAA) were effective in improving preoperative symptoms. On the other hand, 2-year complication rates were higher after AA (27%) than after TAA (16%); however, infection rates were similar (4%). The pub-lished revision rate after AA is 16% versus 11% after TAA. In short, TAA and AA appear to offer the same PROMs, but TAA has a lower rate of com-plications (except for infection) and revisions.

Total Ankle Arthroplasty in Young Patients   53

M. Pierce Ebaugh and William C. McGarvey

> With continuing advancements in total ankle arthroplasty (TAA), it is quickly becoming the procedure of choice for older patients with end-stage ankle arthritis. Multiple studies have been conducted on younger pa-tients who have undergone TAA with promising results, but is it the

procedure of choice? Considerations of TAA versus ankle arthrodesis, TAA implant longevity, outcomes of revision TAA, and whether patients should be offered an arthrodesis with plans for conversion to arthroplasty may help elucidate whether pursuing ankle arthroplasty in a younger, more active population is the correct approach for surgeons.

Outcomes of Lateral Transfibular Approach for Total Ankle Replacement   69

Federico G. Usuelli, Camilla Maccario, and Cristian Indino

Total ankle replacement through a lateral transfibular approach with trabecular metal implants was introduced in 2012 and originally was advertised as a safer approach in terms of wound healing issues. Further studies showed no significant difference comparing anterior and lateral approach for infections and would healing issues, whereas the main advantage is deformity correction, acting on coronal, sagittal, and rotational deformities and on fibular length issues. It showed a survival rate of 97.7% at 5 years follow-up.

Outcomes of Total Ankle Replacement with Preoperative Varus Deformity   81

Laurian J.M. van Es, Daniel Haverkamp, Niek C. van Dijk, and
Laurens W. van der Plaat

Historically, coronal plane deformities of greater than 10° to 15° have been deemed contraindications for total ankle replacement (TAR). However, recent studies show satisfactory results in TAR with severe preoperative varus deformity. When correctly applying ancillary procedures, preoperative varus deformity can be structurally corrected, resulting in similar clinical scores to those obtained with "regular TAR." However, complications and revisions appear to increase with increasing deformity. Unfortunately, results of TAR in varus ankles consist of heterogeneous data (eg, with regards to prosthetic brands, bearing-types, duration of follow-up, and ancillary procedures) precluding strict conclusions. This could be solved by an international consensus group.

Bilateral Total Ankle Arthroplasty   97

Amanda N. Fletcher

Patients with bilateral ankle arthritis have higher rates of primary and secondary/inflammatory arthritis and a more debilitating condition than those with unilateral pathology. The limited bilateral total ankle arthroplasty (TAA) literature supports both 1-surgeon and 2-surgeon team bilateral TAAs as safe and effective with comparable improvements in patient-reported outcome measures (PROMs), complications, reoperations, and prosthesis survival as unilateral TAA and staged bilateral TAA. Additional benefits of bilateral arthroplasty supported in the hip and knee literature include cost reduction, noninferior and even superior perioperative complication profiles, improved PROM and satisfaction, shorter recovery time, early rehabilitation, and less time away from employment.

Outcomes of Total Ankle Arthroplasty After Reoperation due to Gutter Impingement   111

Jaeyoung Kim and Constantine Demetracopoulos

Gutter impingement is one of the most common causes of subsequent surgery after total ankle arthroplasty (TAA). Although gutter debridement has been reported to resolve preoperative symptoms early on, persistent pain after surgery, recurrence, and poor functional outcome scores have been described in patients who have undergone reoperation for gutter debridement. The cause of gutter impingement after TAA is multifactorial, and a better understanding of its causes and optimal surgical techniques for intervention is needed.

Outcomes of Total Ankle Arthroplasty After Periprosthetic Cyst Curettage and Bone Grafting   **123**

Paulo N.F. Ferrao, Nikiforos P. Saragas, and Jaco J. Naude

Total ankle arthroplasty (TAA) has become a popular management option for ankle arthritis. Periprosthetic osteolysis is one of the most common causes for reoperation in TAA. A CT scan should be done in all suspected osteolysis cases to confirm location, quantify size and aid in surgical planning. These patients are often asymptomatic with limited evidence regarding appropriate management. Smaller lesions should be monitored for progression in size. Periprosthetic cysts measuring 10-15mm in all three axes should be considered for debridment and curettage with autogenous bone grafting. The authors believe that bone grafting of large asymptomatic periprosthetic cysts could prevent implant failure.

Diagnosing and Managing Infection in Total Ankle Replacement   **145**

Markus Walther, Veit Krenn, and Kathrin Pfahl

Infections after total ankle replacement (TAR) within the first 4 weeks after implantation can be managed successfully with 1 or several debridements, irrigation, and a change of polyethylene inlay. Late infections require implant removal. Low-grade infections might be an underestimated problem so far. Although single-surgery revisions are reported in the literature, the authors' experience with 2-stage revisions using an antibiotics-loaded bone cement spacer is better. Additional antibiotics are used to support the surgical treatment. After antibiotic therapy of 12 weeks, the final treatment includes ankle or tibio-talo-calcaneal fusion and, with limitations, revision TAR.

Complications in Total Ankle Replacement   **157**

Joris P.S. Hermus

The debate between ankle arthrodesis and total ankle replacement for patients with end-stage arthritis of the ankle joint is an ongoing topic in orthopedic surgery. Ankle arthrodesis, or fusion, has been the traditional treatment for ankle arthritis. It involves fusing the bones of the ankle joint together, eliminating the joint and creating a solid bony union. Arthrodesis is effective in reducing pain in the ankle, but it results in a loss of ankle motion. This can increase the load on adjacent joints, such as the subtalar joint, which may lead to accelerated degeneration and arthritis in those joints over time.

Outcomes of Conversion of Ankle Fusion to Total Ankle Arthroplasty   **165**

Christopher Traynor and J. Chris Coetzee

With ankle replacements gaining popularity and documented good functional outcomes, there is an increasing number of patients inquiring about the possibility of converting an ankle fusion to a replacement. This could be due to pain, limited function, or increasing adjacent joint arthritis. There is an increasing body of evidence in the literature that a conversion to a replacement is possible and that the outcomes are positive. There are also absolute contradictions for a conversion. An absent fibula, pain of unknown origin, and recent infection fall in this category. Long-term follow-up is needed to see if conversions of ankle fusions to replacements have the same functional results and longevity as primary replacements.

Outcomes of Revision Total Ankle Replacement   **171**

Bakur A. Jamjoom and Sunil Dhar

The objective of this study is to provide an up-to-date review of the outcomes of revision total ankle arthroplasty (TAA). Relevant studies published over the last decade were reviewed. Twelve studies were included. At a median follow-up of 4 years, the median survival and reoperation rates were 86% and 16%, respectively. Significant postoperative improvements in patient-reported outcome measures were recorded in 6 studies. Significant improvement in alignment was documented in 1 study only. Revision TAA is a safe procedure that can produce good outcomes. Nevertheless, data relating to long-term outcome are still limited in quantity and duration.

FOOT AND ANKLE CLINICS

FORTHCOMING ISSUES

June 2024
Osteochondral Lesions of the Foot and Ankle
Camilla Maccario, *Editor*

September 2024
Updates in Hallux Rigidus
James Albert Nunley, *Editor*

December 2024
Pathology of the Lesser Toes
Caio Nery, *Editor*

RECENT ISSUES

December 2023
Innovative Approaches on Cavovarus Deformity: Thinking Outside of the Box
Alessio Bernasconi, *Editor*

September 2023
Advanced Imaging of the Foot and Ankle
Jan Fritz, *Editor*

June 2023
Complexities Involving the Ankle Sprain
Alexandre Leme Godoy-Santos, *Editor*

RELATED SERIES

Orthopedic Clinics
Clinics in Sports Medicine
Physical Medicine and Rehabilitation Clinics

THE CLINICS ARE NOW AVAILABLE ONLINE!
Access your subscription at:
www.theclinics.com

FOOT AND ANKLE CLINICS

FORTHCOMING ISSUES

June 2024
Osteochondral Lesions of the Foot and
Ankle
Camilla Maccario, Editor

September 2024
Updates in Hallux Rigidus
James A Nunley II, Editor

December 2024
Pathology of the Lesser Toes
Caio Nery, Editor

RECENT ISSUES

December 2023
Innovative Approaches on Cavovarus
Deformity: Thinking Outside of the Box
Alessio Bernasconi, Editor

September 2023
Advanced Imaging of the Foot and Ankle
Jan Fritz, Editor

June 2023
Complexities involving the Ankle Sprain
Alexandre Leme Godoy-Santos, Editor

RELATED SERIES

Orthopedic Clinics
Clinics in Sports Medicine
Physical Medicine and Rehabilitation Clinics

Preface

What You Will Find in this Collection of Current Total Ankle Arthroplasty Articles

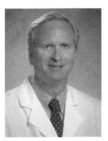

Mark E. Easley, MD
Editor

I am honored that Cesar asked me to serve as guest editor. My Duke colleagues and I continue to advance the practice and science of total ankle arthroplasty (TAA), and our original work is frequently enhanced through our review of the experience and research of other investigators dedicated to improving the lives of their patients with end-stage ankle arthritis. I am privileged to present this collection of articles written by a talented group of international experts in TAA. I am thankful to them for agreeing to participate in this meaningful educational endeavor, and I am humbled by their excellent contributions. These surgeons not only share their clinical experience in primary, revision, and complex TAA but also provide objective and critical analysis of total ankle outcomes. I am confident that this issue will serve as a valuable resource for you to optimize your management of ankle arthritis.

Conflict of interest/disclosures: Consultant, Royalties Exactech.

Mark E. Easley, MD
Duke Foot and Ankle Service
Duke University Health System
2812 Chelsea Circle
Durham, NC 27707, USA

Foot Ankle Clin N Am 29 (2024) xv
https://doi.org/10.1016/j.fcl.2023.09.008
1083-7515/24/© 2023 Published by Elsevier Inc.

foot.theclinics.com

Preface

What You Will Find in this Collection of Current Total Ankle Arthroplasty Articles

Quality of Outcomes Research in Total Ankle Arthroplasty

Kamran Hamid, MD, MPH[a], Ryan LeDuc, MD[a],*

KEYWORDS

- Total ankle arthroplasty • Ankle arthroplasty • Ankle replacement
- Outcomes research

KEY POINTS

- Total ankle arthroplasty (TAA) has gained increasing interest, largely due to improved outcomes demonstrated through short- and mid-term research for newer, third-generation implant designs.
- Initial first-generation implants were abandoned due to high rates of bone loss, osteolysis, wound-related issues, and implant-associated complications.
- Enthusiasm for TAA in the treatment of end-stage ankle arthritis must be tempered by quality research with longer follow-up and a high level of evidence.

INTRODUCTION, HISTORY, DEFINITIONS, AND BACKGROUND

Total ankle arthroplasty (TAA) has gained increasing interest, largely due to improved outcomes demonstrated through short- and mid-term research for newer, third-generation implant designs. Initial first-generation implants were abandoned due to high rates of bone loss, osteolysis, wound-related issues, and implant-associated complications.[1–5] Second-generation implants sought to address several issues encountered with the early designs and introduced porous, metal-backed surfaces. Despite improved implant osseointegration and less osteolysis, the second-generation implants demonstrated high rates of polyethylene wear, impingement, implant subsidence/migration, and syndesmotic nonunion (Agility prosthesis).[6] Third-generation and fourth-generation implant systems feature designs and surgical techniques that require afford less bone resection and improved bony ingrowth compared with earlier generation implants. Improvements in implant design, surgical technique and

[a] Department of Orthopaedic Surgery, Loyola University Medical Center, 2160 South First Avenue, c/o Sonia Raigoza, Orthopaedic Surgery, Maywood, IL 60153, USA
* Corresponding author. 2160 South First Avenue, Maguire Building Suite 1700, Maywood, IL 60153, USA
E-mail address: Ryan.LeDuc@luhs.org

Foot Ankle Clin N Am 29 (2024) 1–9
https://doi.org/10.1016/j.fcl.2023.09.001
1083-7515/24/© 2023 Elsevier Inc. All rights reserved.
foot.theclinics.com

instrumentation have broadened indications for TAA to include ankle arthritis with deformity and/or marked bone loss.

Enthusiasm for TAA in the treatment of end-stage ankle arthritis must be tempered by quality research with longer follow-up and a high level of evidence (LOE). In a review of TAA design rationale, Gross and colleagues caution that favorable early outcomes may succumb to poor mid- to long-term follow-up.[7] Fortunately, careful follow-up of third- and fourth-generation implants suggests that favorable early results may be maintained at longer follow-up.

Perhaps even more important than TAA results is evidence-based research quality. In our current medical environment, rising health care costs demand high-quality clinical research to support patients' proposed treatment plans. The term "evidence-based medicine" was introduced in 1991.[8] Twelve years later, the Journal of Bone and Joint Surgery (JBJS) began assigning a LOE score of its published research, with the intent to improve the scientific process and indicate a study's quality.[9,10] The LOE score identifies criteria for study methodology, analysis, and statistical methods, thereby allowing the reader to weigh the significance of the study results and their clinical relevance. In 2008, *Foot and Ankle International* (FAI) and *Journal of Foot and Ankle Surgery* similarly implemented assigning levels of evidence to the published literature (**Fig. 1**). Several review articles have assessed the LOE in the orthopedic literature, with some focused in foot and ankle.[11–15] A concerning conclusion from these review articles is that clinical decision-making is often based on the conclusion of published literature assigned a low LOE (III, IV, or V).

Our purpose was to assess the quality of outcomes research in TAA. In a recent review article, our senior author and colleagues presented the quality of outcomes research in TAA through 2019.[14] The authors suggested using the collective experience of hip and knee arthroplasty surgeons as a model. Through rigorous study designs and assessment of evidence, biases in the literature were limited. Moreover, complications associated with trends in hip and knee arthroplasty were more readily identified, and appropriate changes were made to address these shortcomings.

Several epidemiologic studies detail the increase in TAA in recent years.[16,17] Shah and colleagues noted that the incidence of TAA is projected to continue to rapidly rise over the next decade.[17] From 2005 to 2017, the United States experienced a 564% increase in primary TAA. The projections of this study estimate an additional increase up to 796% by the year 2030 (**Figs. 2** and **3**). Commensurate with the increasing TAA case volume is the amount of dedicated TAA with longer term follow-up become

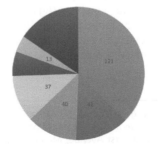

FAI   JBJS   Foot Ankle Surg   Journal Foot Ankle   BJJ   Foot Ankle Specialist   Other

Fig. 1. Publications by Journal. The number of outcomes studies published by journal from 2006 to 2022. *Foot and Ankle International* (FAI) was the most frequently used journal; 61.2% of articles were published in a foot and ankle specific journal, whereas the remaining 28.8% were published in either a general orthopedic journal or journal of another category.

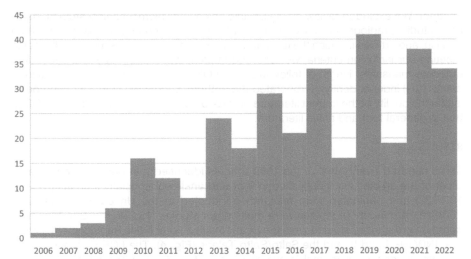

Fig. 2. Number of publications by year. The annual incidence of new publications is recorded. As demonstrated, there has been a trend toward an increasing number of publications by year over the past 16 years, which has been sustained in more recent years.

available for review. Our review incorporates a vastly broader amount of research available for careful assessment of the quality of TAA research.

OUR METHODS OF ASSESSING RELEVANT OUTCOMES RESEARCH

We identified all peer-reviewed, English-language TAA outcomes studies between January 2006 and December 2022. Initially, we searched PubMed for the terms "total ankle arthroplasty" and "total ankle replacement" and reviewed all results by title and

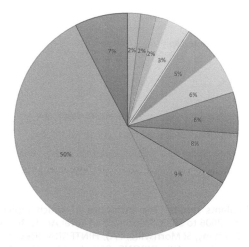

■ France ■ Netherlands ■ Japan ■ Germany ■ Canada ■ UK ■ Italy ■ Switzerland ■ South Korea ■ US ■ Other

Fig. 3. Publications by country. The proportion of the publications published in individual countries. For the publications that qualified for this review, one-half were published in the United States.

abstract. We excluded review articles, basic science or biomechanical studies, database studies, radiographic assessments, articles published in a language other than English, and articles in which the full manuscript could not be accessed. For all articles meeting our inclusion criteria, we recorded implant type, all primary and secondary outcome measures, length of follow-up, and LOE. To confirm cited LOE, our senior author (KH) independently corroborated the authors' suggested LOE. Our hypothesis is that the quality of the current literature on TAA outcomes in TAA has a similar LOE to that in general foot and ankle literature.

RESULTS

Three hundred twenty-two of the 1599 articles identified met our inclusion criteria. Most of the articles were published in foot and ankle subspecialty journals (61.2%, 197/322) and originated from research conducted in the United States (49.6%, 160/322). A minority of studies were multicenter studies (15.2%, 49/322). The most common prostheses studied were the Scandinavian Total Ankle Replacement, Hintegra, INBONE I and II, and the Salto/Salto Talaris (**Fig. 4**). The LOE assigned by the authors or respective journal is summarized in **Fig. 5**; over one-fourth of articles were not assigned an LOE by the authors and/or journal. Most of the studies (27.6% and 39.4%, respectively) had Level III evidence (27.6%) or Level IV evidence (39.4%), with the most common study design being case series (64.9%, 209/322). We reviewed far more retrospective investigations (81.4%) than prospective investigations (18.6%). Only two randomized control trials were identified. Patient-reported outcome measurements varied, with the most commonly used assessment tools being the American Orthopedic Foot and Ankle Society (AOFAS) score (153/322) and the pain visual analog scale (138/322). Across all studies, average mean follow-up was 49 months (standard deviation [STD], ± 40), average minimum follow-up was 27.6 months (STD, ± 25) months, and average maximum follow-up was 70 months (STD, ± 50).

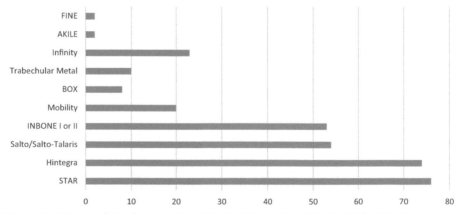

Fig. 4. Incidence of implants studies. The incidence in which individual implants were named in the studies from 2006 to 2022. Scandinavian Total Ankle Replacement (STAR; Waldemar Link, Hamburg, Germany; Si Morrisville, PA), HINTEGRA. (Newsteal SA, Lyon, France), Salto-Talaris (Integra, Plainsboro, NJ), INBONE (Wright Medical, Memphis, TN), Infinity (Wright Medical, Memphis, TN), Zimmer Trabecular Metal (ZTM; Zimmer Biomet, Warsaw, IN), Mobility (gePuy, Warsaw, IN), Bologna-Oxford (BOX; MatOrtho, Leatherhead, Surrey, UK), AKILE (Lavender Medical, Stevenage, UK), FINE (FINE; Nakashima Medical Company, Okayama, Japan).

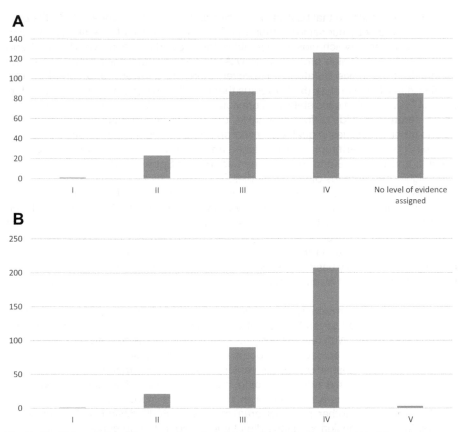

Fig. 5. (*A, B*) Level of evidence assigned and by independent assessment. Discrepancy was noted between the level of evidence assigned by the article writers and by independent assessment. A higher proportion of studies were of Levels III and IV evidence on independent assessment than what was reported by the article authors/journals.

DISCUSSION

Accurately assessing the quality of outcomes research is important. Numerous factors determine whether a study is high quality, including study design/type, methodology, and statistical analysis. As providers we are inundated with a new research that influences accepted clinical decision-making algorithms and we need to identify high-quality research that is most impactful. The American Academy of Orthopedic Surgeons (AAOS) releases Clinical Practice Guidelines (CPGs), described as "evidence-based programs for current orthopedic diagnostic, treatment, and postoperative procedures" (AAOS, Rosemont, IL; AAOS.org). These CPGs are based on an up-to-date assessment of the body of literature and demonstrate how assessing the quality of research can be used to influence practice habits.

Our review aims to provide an updated overview of the quality of research in the published TAA literature. We found that the quality of TAA literature reflects the reported quality of the general body of foot and ankle literature, though with some slight differences and limitations. Barske and colleagues reported on the quality of research and LOE in the foot and ankle literature in 2010; they found that 66% were Level IV, 15% were Level III, and 12% were Level II. When stratifying trends for individual journals, they observed that 63% of FAI articles were level IV evidence.[11] Over the past 16 years, a study by our senior author (KH) found that 64.3% of TAA studies were of Level IV evidence, which closely resembles the proportion seen overall in foot and ankle literature.[14] A high proportion of TAA studies compare their outcomes to the general foot and ankle literature.[13] However, there are a lower proportion of Level II studies in the TAA literature (6.5%) versus that reported in general foot and ankle literature (17%), a finding consistent with previous reports.[14] When compared with orthopedic literature outside of foot and ankle, the overall TAA literature remains slightly behind other specialties in quality of research and LOE. Published literature suggests that the Journal of Arthroplasty's published articles are 13% Level I studies and 17% Level II, and the JBJS and the American Journal of Sports Medicine have reported even higher percentages of Level I studies.[10]

Level IV studies, despite their lower quality, may prove to be of value and contribute to the literature. We maintain that Level IV studies add value to the body of evidence and that meaningful conclusions may be gleaned from these studies. Provided that results reported in Level IV studies are interpreted with the knowledge that there may be inherent biases in these study designs, lower quality retrospective studies may represent the only basis for providers to determine best clinical practices. In addition, results from Level IV retrospective studies may prompt higher quality prospective randomized trials.

As pointed out by previously by our senior author (KH), TAA is a relatively novel procedure that has seen several waves of utilization with the advent of newer implant design generations. With few exceptions, TAA is typically performed at many higher volume institutions by surgeons with dedicated training in TAA and potential conflicts. In his previously published study, our senior author reported that through 2019, 10% of TAA studies disclosed industry funding, but an additional 28% failed to report their funding source. This is a relatively high proportion of industry-sponsored studies, which introduces another potential area of bias in study design and reporting of results. Moreover, design surgeons directly involved in the outcomes research may bias study results and their validity.

In our opinion, the learning curve for TAA is relevant to the study of outcomes. Several authors compared complication rates in "early" and "late" patient cohorts.[18–24] Roukis and Simonson's systematic review suggested an overall complication rate of 44.2% in the learning curve phase, described as "during initial performance of primary total ankle arthroplasty." Based on two commonly used classification schemes, 10.3% were considered high-grade complications, 19.3% were medium grade, and 54.2% were low grade.[24] Panchbhavi and colleagues defined a high-volume TAA arthroplasty surgeon as one who performs 11 or more TAAs annually. As of 2015, there were only 53 surgeons in the United States who fulfilled this definition of a high-volume TAA surgeon.[25] Although we do not have current access to individual surgeon volume, we suspect that a large proportion of TAA research is published by high-volume surgeons. We maintain that TAA results published by experienced, high-volume (and design-team) TAA surgeons should not commensurate with the results routinely expected or reported for the majority of practicing orthopedic surgeons. Although this does not necessarily indicate that the TAA literature is systemically flawed, this may be a consideration when discussing the generalizability of the results of these studies and attempting to extrapolate the outcomes to the average orthopedic surgeon.

With regard to the most commonly used patient-reported outcome measurement tools, the AOFAS hindfoot-ankle score was the most commonly used measurement tool. The AOFAS score was found in nearly half of the reviewed publications (153/322). The AOFAS score was developed in 1994 by the AOFAS to provide a standard method for reporting the clinical status of the ankle and foot. Although the AOFAS score is not validated, it continues to be widely adopted in foot and ankle literature to quantify clinical status. The score considers both subjective and objective data points to draw data and describe function, alignment, and pain.[26] Many other patient-reported outcome measurement tools were identified in our review, and Hannan and colleagues provide a succinct summary of several of these patient-reported outcomes measurement (PROM) tools.[27]

A potential area of criticism of the body of evidence for TAA literature is that the mean follow-up in all of the TAA studies we reviewed was limited to 49 months. We recognize the relative novelty of third- and fourth-generation implants and the recent increase in their utilization and that the majority of published TAA studies published only include short- to mid-term follow-up data. We only identified select studies with longer term follow-up and maintain that we need continued investigation of existing patient cohorts and new prospective, randomized comparative trials to accurately assess survivorship, quality, and functional outcomes of TAA.

We acknowledge the challenges inherent to the study of TAA, especially when compared with the study of total hip and/or total knee arthroplasty, challenges that our senior author previously published.[14] First, end-stage ankle arthritis is rare relative to hip and knee arthritis, with the prevalence of ankle arthritis estimated at 1% of the population.[28,29] Doctors' office visits for hip and knee arthritis are far more common than are those for ankle arthritis, with some studies suggesting 9 to 10 times more common.[28,30,31] Given the large discrepancy, the volume of hip and knee arthroplasty that of TAA. Furthermore, unlike for the hip and knee, ankle arthrodesis continues to be a common alternative in the surgical management of end-stage ankle arthritis.[32,33]

SUMMARY

The study of outcomes in TAA is a topic that has gained increasing interest recently, and this update demonstrates a continuation in the trend in a steady increase. Most of the publications on TAA involve retrospective study with short- to mid-term follow-up. In addition, the patient-reported outcomes measurement tools used vary in the literature, though the most commonly used tool is the nonvalidated AOFAS score. Although outcomes research on ankle replacement certainly does have its pitfalls, the results of the current literature are nonetheless useful to those who perform TAA as they provide early recognition of adverse events and poorly performing implants. These studies also provide direction on where future research efforts should focus in order. Of note, long-term outcomes studies would further improve the overall quality of the research as a whole, as would adoption of a more standardized, validated PROM tool. Last, no surgeon database of TAA exists to the authors' knowledge. Having a standardized database for reporting outcomes data would be beneficial as the incidence of TAA, while growing consistently over the past 2 decades, is still relatively small, which leads to difficulty in properly powering well-designed studies.

CLINICS CARE POINTS

- Total ankle arthroplasty (TAA) utilization is sharply increasing due to newer generation implant designs, improved instrumentation, and a better understanding of reasons for failure.
- Outcomes research in TAA has increased as well over the past 16 years.

- Most of the outcomes studies on the topic remain lower level of evidence studies, with very few randomized control trials assessing efficacy and outcomes of TAA.
- Patient-reported outcomes measurement tools are varied, and the most commonly used tool is a nonvalidated scoring system.
- Although the improved outcomes noted on retrospective studies, well-designed, higher level of evidence studies are needed.

DISCLOSURE

The authors of this article have no disclosures to report.

REFERENCES

1. Cracchiolo A III, DeOrio JK. Design features of current total ankle replacements: Implants and instrumentation. J Am Acad Orthop Surg 2008;16(9):530–40.
2. Bolton-Maggs BG, Sudlow RA, Freeman MA. Total ankle arthroplasty: A long-term review of the London Hospital experience. J Bone Joint Surg Br 1985;67(5): 785–90.
3. Newton SE. An artificial ankle joint. Clin Orthop Relat Res 1979;142:141–5.
4. Pappas M, Buechel FF, DePalma AF. Cylindrical total ankle joint replacement: Surgical and biomechanical rationale. Clin Orthop Relat Res 1976;118:82–92.
5. Vickerstaff JA, Miles AW, Cunningham JL. A brief history of total ankle replacement and a review of the current status. Med Eng Phys 2007;29(10):1056–64.
6. Thomas RH, Daniels TR. Ankle arthritis. J Bone Joint Surg Am 2003;85(5):923–36.
7. Gross C, Palanca A, DeOrio J. Design Rationale for Total Ankle Arthroplasty Systems: An Update. J Am Acad Orthop Surg 2018;26(10):353–9.
8. Guyatt GH. Evidence-based medicine. ACP J Club 1991;114. A–16.
9. Wright JG, Swiontkowski MF, Heckman JD. Introducing levels of evidence to the journal. J Bone Joint Surg Am 2003;85(1):1–3. PMID: 12533564.
10. Obremsky W, Pappas N, Attalah-Wasif E, et al. Level of evidence in orthoapedic journals. J Bone Joint Surg Am 2005;87:2632–8.
11. Barske HL, Baumhauer J. Quality of research and level of evidence in foot and ankle publications. FAI 2012;33:1–6.
12. Sugrue CM, Joyce CW, Sugrue RM, et al. Trends in the level of evidence in clinical hand surgery. Hand 2016;11:211–5.
13. Turlik MA, Kushner D. Levels of evidence of articles in podiatric medical journals. J Am Podiatr Med Assoc 2000;90:300–2.
14. Foran IM, Vafek EC, Bohl DD, et al. Quality Assessment of Modern Total Ankle Arthroplasty Clinical Outcomes Research. J Foot Ankle Surg 2022;61(1):7–11.
15. Shah NS, Umeda Y, Suriel Peguero E, et al. Outcome Reporting in Total Ankle Arthroplasty: A Systematic Review. J Foot Ankle Surg 2021;60(4):770–6.
16. Karzon AL, Kadakia RJ, Coleman MM, et al. The Rise of Total Ankle Arthroplasty Use: A Database Analysis Describing Case Volumes and Incidence Trends in the United States Between 2009 and 2019. Foot Ankle Int 2022;43(11):1501–10.
17. Shah JA, Schwartz AM, Farley KX, et al. Projections and Epidemiology of Total Ankle and Revision Total Ankle Arthroplasty in the United States to 2030 [published online ahead of print, 2022 Jul 14]. Foot Ankle Spec 2022. 193864002211 09420.
18. Myerson MS, Mroczek K. Perioperative complications of total ankle arthroplasty. Foot Ankle Int 2003;24:17–21.

19. Haskell A, Mann RA. Perioperative complication rate of total ankle replacement is reduced by surgeon experience. Foot Ankle Int 2004;25:283–9.
20. Kumar A, Dhar S. Total ankle replacement: early results during learning period. Foot Ankle Surg 2007;13:19–23.
21. Lee KB, Cho SG, Hur CI, et al. Perioperative complications of Hintegra total ankle replacement: our initial 50 cases. Foot Ankle Int 2008;29:978–84.
22. Saltzman CL, Mann RA, Ahrens JE, et al. Prospective controlled trial of STAR total ankle replacement versus ankle fusion: initial results. Foot Ankle Int 2009;30: 579–96.
23. Lee KT, Lee YK, Young KW, et al. Perioperative complications and learning curve of the Mobility total ankle system. Foot Ankle Int 2013;34:210–4.
24. Simonson DC, Roukis TS. Incidence of Complications During the Surgeon Learning Curve Period for Primary Total Ankle Replacement: A Systematic Review. Clin Podiatr Med Surg 2015;32(4):473–82.
25. Stein B, Somerson J, Janney C, et al. Distribution of High-Volume Ankle Replacement Surgeons in United States Metropolitan Areas. Foot Ankle Spec 2022;15(2): 127–35.
26. Kitaoka HB, Alexander IJ, Adelaar RS, et al. Clinical rating systems for the ankle-hindfoot, midfoot, hallux, and lesser toes. Foot Ankle Int 1994;15(7):349–53.
27. Riskowski JL, Hagedorn TJ, Hannan MT. Measures of foot function, foot health, and foot pain: American Academy of Orthopedic Surgeons Lower Limb Outcomes Assessment: Foot and Ankle Module (AAOS-FAM), Bristol Foot Score (BFS), Revised Foot Function Index (FFI-R), Foot Health Status Questionnaire (FHSQ), Manchester Foot Pain and Disability Index (MFPDI), Podiatric Health Questionnaire (PHQ), and Rowan Foot Pain Assessment (ROFPAQ). Arthritis Care Res 2011;63(Suppl 11):S229–39.
28. Huch K, Kuettner KE, Dieppe P. Osteoarthritis in ankle and knee joints. Semin Arthritis Rheum 1997;26(4):667–74.
29. Valderrabano V, Horisberger M, Russell I, et al. Etiology of ankle osteoarthritis. Clin Orthop Relat Res 2009;467(7):1800–6.
30. Buckwalter JA, Saltzman C, Brown T. The impact of osteoarthritis: implications for research. Clin Orthop Relat Res 2004;427(Suppl):S6–15.
31. Cushnaghan J, Dieppe P. Study of 500 patients with limb joint osteoarthritis. I. Analysis by age, sex, and distribution of symptomatic joint sites. Ann Rheum Dis 1991;50(1):8–13.
32. Harkess JW and Crockarell JR. Chapter 3: Arthroplasty of the hip, In: Canale ST and Beaty JH, Campbell's operative orthopaedics, 12th edition, 2013, Elsevier Mosby, Philadelphia, PA, 166-311.
33. Mihalko WM. Chapter 7: Arthroplasty of the knee, In: Canale ST and Beaty JH, Campbell's operative orthopaedics, 12th edition, 2013, Elsevier Mosby, Philadelphia, PA, 396-468.

Clinical Outcomes and Registry Data in Total Ankle Arthroplasty

Kenneth J. Hunt, MD*, Daniel Ross, MD, Francisco Fontan, MD

KEYWORDS

- Ankle arthroplasty • Total ankle replacement • Ankle arthritis • Registry
- Patient-reported outcomes

KEY POINTS

- Total ankle arthroplasty (TAA) is an effective treatment for end-stage ankle arthritis consistently demonstrating good to excellent outcomes.
- There is little consensus on preferred patient-reported outcome metrics (PROMs) for assessing outcomes.
- Several countries have successful registries to track longevity of TAA in populations; however, PROMs are generally not successfully tracked in registries.
- A trend toward consensus on outcome metrics and collaborative registries is warranted to optimize patient selection and outcomes in TAA.

INTRODUCTION

Total ankle arthroplasty (TAA) is a highly effective treatment for end-stage ankle arthritis, providing pain relief and good functional results at follow-up.[1] Increasingly, investigators are reporting good outcomes and high satisfaction rates, leading to increased interest in ankle arthroplasty in the past decade as an alternative to ankle fusion.[2] This has also led to a relatively rapid evolution of new implants, material improvements on existing implants, and debate regarding which outcome metrics are best to truly evaluate success following ankle arthroplasty. Further, because ankle replacements are still much less common that hip and knee replacements, high-volume centers, and large data registries are less common and less populated for TAA.

Compounding the challenge in understanding clinical outcomes following TAA is the lack of uniformity in patient-reported outcome metrics (PROMs) when tracking and describing clinical outcomes from the patient perspective. Much of this stems from an orthopedic ankle specialty transition away from the American Orthopedic Foot

Department of Orthopaedic Surgery, University of Colorado School of Medicine, 12631 East 17th Avenue, Room 4508, Aurora, CO 80045, USA
* Corresponding author.
E-mail address: KENNETH.J.HUNT@CUANSCHUTZ.EDU

Foot Ankle Clin N Am 29 (2024) 11–26
https://doi.org/10.1016/j.fcl.2023.09.006
1083-7515/24/© 2023 Elsevier Inc. All rights reserved.

and Ankle Society (AOFAS) scales[3] and toward the Patient Reported Outcomes Measurement Information System (PROMIS) scales.[4] Still, there is a need for a consistent ankle-specific subscale that is not currently met. This article explores the PROMs used to describe the results of TAA and an overview of existing national TAA registries.

IMPLANTS, PATIENT-REPORTED OUTCOME METRICS, AND FOLLOW-UP IN TOTAL ANKLE ARTHROPLASTY CLINICAL OUTCOME STUDIES

A collection of validated patient-reported outcome (PRO) surveys from orthopedic patients has been available since the early 1990s and are increasingly used in both clinical care and outcomes research. Despite several PROMs validated for ankle arthritis, there is no present consensus on the best PROM to use when following these patients. Using the PubMed database, we performed a search for all English language peer-reviewed studies regarding TAA PROs from January 2010 to May 2023. Our initial search included terms "total ankle arthroplasty outcomes," and "total ankle replacement outcomes." We excluded articles that did not include PROs. We also excluded articles solely focusing on implants that are no longer commercially available (eg, Mobility Total Ankle Replacement, Depuy, Leeds, UK or Agility Total Ankle, Depuy, Warsaw, IN, USA). However, articles assessing a pooled mix of available and unavailable implants were included. We further excluded duplicate articles, articles focusing on total talus replacement, national registry articles, and articles where the complete text was not available. After exclusions, we identified 173 articles which are included in the writing of this article. Of these, 155 articles were cohort or comparison studies, with 18 systematic reviews or meta-analysis. Owing to reference constraints in this publication, only the most recent and relevant publications are included.

A total of 27 unique PROMs were used in TAA outcomes studies. The most used PROs were the AOFAS score (47% of articles), the Visual Analog Scale (VAS) (43.3%), and the 36-Item Short Form Survey (SF-36) (32%) (**Fig. 1**). These frequencies are similar to previously rates of PRO usage.[5]

For clinical outcome studies, the United States published the largest percent (42.5%), followed by European countries (24.5%), Canada (14.2%), Asian countries (10.3%), and the United Kingdom (6.5%) (**Fig. 2**). These findings are consistent with previously published rates of article origin countries.[6]

Within the included studies, 23 different TAA implants were used. The Scandinavian Total Ankle Replacement (STAR, Don Joy Orthopedics, Lewisville, TX, USA) was the most frequently included (35.2%), followed by the HINTEGRA (Integra LifeSciences,

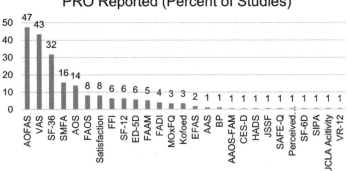

Fig. 1. Percent of clinical outcome studies reporting on each PRO.

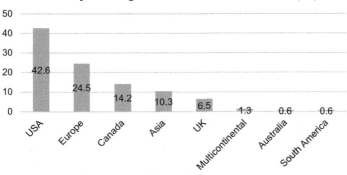

Fig. 2. Country of origin for published of PRO studies.

Plainsboro, New Jersey, USA) (31.8%), and SALTO-TALARIS (Smith & Nephew, Memphis, TN, USA) (23.7%). Multiple articles (10.4%) did not list specific implant type, or simply listed "other" (2.3%) (**Fig. 3**).

The average patient follow-up in TAA studies is 52.6 months (range 12–188.8 months). There is no consensus on the definitions of "short-term," "midterm," and "long-term" follow-up for orthopedic literature. In a 2021 systematic review by Ahmad and colleagues,[7] the investigators proposed that follow-up periods of less than 30 months (<2.5 years), 30 to 150 months (2.5–12.5 years), and greater than 150 months (>12.5 years) define short term, midterm, and long term, respectively. By these criteria, there are 35 short-term follow-up studies, 121 midterm follow-up, and only three long-term follow-up studies. In 14 articles, the follow-up timing was not specified or could not be determined. **Fig. 4** further subdivides midterm into "early" midterm (30–90 months) and "late" midterm (90–150 months). Most of the published studies detail short- or early midterm follow-up, with few studies assessing TAA PROs beyond 12.5 years.

TAA outcome studies generally report based on a variety of criteria and comparisons (**Fig. 5**). The most common criterion is the implant (40.5%), Criteria 1. This is followed by comparison of TAA versus ankle arthrodesis (AA) (21.7%) Criteria 2, revision TAA (RTAA) surgery (6.9%) Criteria 3, TAA in coronal deformity (5.8%) Criteria 4, TAA in hemophilia patients (4.6%) Criteria 5, patient age (2.9%) Criteria 6, and bilateral TAA surgeries

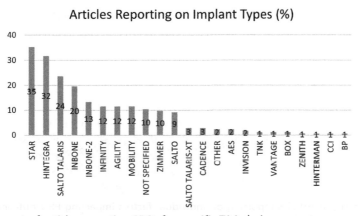

Fig. 3. Percent of articles reporting PROs for specific TAA designs.

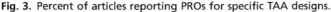

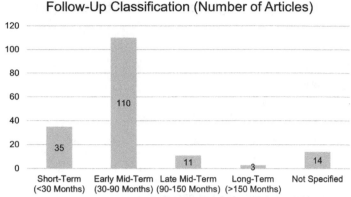

Fig. 4. Classification of follow-up duration for published studies.

(3.4%) Criteria 7. These findings are consistent with prior published reports on investigational topics.[5] Five articles covered multiple topics in their respective studies.

Criteria 1: Outcomes of Specific Implants

In the below section, we will provide an overview of the published follow-up, survivorship, and PRO results for the more commonly investigated implants, still currently available on the market. Of note, the vast majority of current TAA implants have received FDA clearance in the past 10 years, so there is limited long-term follow-up.

Scandinavian Total Ankle Replacement

The STAR (Don Joy Orthopedics, Lewisville, TX, USA) is the implant with most clinical studies reporting PROs (60 studies). For studies reporting patient follow-up, the average was 61.2 months (12–188.4 months). The STAR implant demonstrates high survivorship in early follow-up studies (94%–96%).[8] There is a wider range for midterm follow-up (78%–100%)[9,10] and a measurable decrease in survivorship for studies reporting beyond 10 years (63.6%–87.8%).[11,12]

In early follow-up studies, the STAR implant demonstrates consistent improvement in PROs from preoperative measurements.[13–15] Scott and colleagues[15] demonstrated significant improvements in SF-36, VAS, and AOFAS scores at 12 months. Cunningham

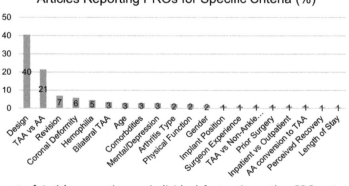

Fig. 5. Percent of Articles reporting on individual factors impacting PRO outcomes in patients undergoing TAA.

and colleagues[14] likewise reported improvements in SF-36, VAS, and short musculo-skeletal function assessment (SMFA) scores. Another study showed a decrease in pain (VAS), improvements in AOFAS and SF-36 regardless of age at 27.6 months.[16]

At midterm follow-up, the STAR implant has likewise performed well, demonstrating significant improvements in VAS, SF-36, AOFAS, buechel pappas (BP), foot function index (FFI), Kofoed, and Ankle Osteoarthritis Scale (AOS) scores.[10,17–20] At long-term follow-up, the STAR implant maintains significant improvement in PROs including AOFAS, Kofoed, VAS, BP, FFI, and EQ-5D with high satisfaction rates, despite the drop-off in survivorship as noted above.[11,21–23]

HINTEGRA

The HINTEGRA (Integra LifeSciences, Plainsboro, New Jersey, USA) was reported in 55 articles investigating PROs. The average reported follow-up for these studies 61.5 months (24–115.2 months). Early survivorship has been documented as high as 91%–100%[24–26] and midterm survivorship of 76%–100%.[27–31] At longer follow-up, survivorship is reported as 81.2%–93.5%.[32–34]

Early follow-up studies demonstrate improvements in AOFAS, VAS, SF-36, CES-D, and SF-12 scores.[25,35,36] These improvements are seen regardless of gender,[36] bilateral versus unilateral TAA surgeries,[37] preoperative depressed state,[35] and final implant position.[25] At midterm follow-up, the HINTEGRA implant further shows positive improvements on PROs including AOFAS, VAS, University of California at Los Angeles (UCLA) activity score, SF-36, and AOS,[26,27,38–43] with high satisfaction.[26] Studies with the longest follow-up reporting on HINTEGRA demonstrate maintained improvements in patient satisfaction, AOFAS, VAS, and AOS scores.[32–34]

SALTO-TALARIS

The SALTO-TALARIS (Smith & Nephew, Memphis, TN, USA), was investigated in 41 studies focusing on PROs. Patient follow-up was reported in 40 studies, with an average of 43.8 months (19.2–85.2 months). At early follow-up survivorship is reported as 98.1% to 99%.[44,45] Midterm follow-up demonstrated survivorship of 95.6%–97.5%.[46,47] With the longest average follow-up reported at 85.2 months,[46] there were no late-term clinical outcome studies included.

In early follow-up, the SALTO-TALARIS implant has demonstrated improved clinical outcome scores from preoperative assessments.[14,45,47–50] In their 2-year follow-up study of 109 SALTO-TALARIS implants, Hendy and colleagues[44] reported improvements in all measured PROs including VAS, Foot and Ankle Ability Measure (FAAM) (Activities of Daily Living [ADL] and Sports), and SF-12. When compared with competitor implants, at early follow-up, the SALTO-TALARIS implant demonstrated similar improvements in outcomes including AOFAS, SMFA, VAS, SF-36, and Foot and Ankle Disability Index (FADI) in multiple studies.[13,51] At midterm follow-up, studies have shown consistent improvements in PROs.[46,52]

INBONE and INBONE-II

The INBONE and INBONE-II Total Ankle Systems (Wright Medical/Stryker, Memphis, TN, USA) were investigated in 48 PRO studies combined (average follow-up 43.8 months, range 15.4–98.4 months). Sixteen studies included on INBONE, 23 of these studies included INBONE-II, and 8 reported on both.

High early survivorship was demonstrated for both implants by Lewis and colleagues, with 94% for INBONE and 97.4% for INBONE-II at 25.2 months.[53] In midterm studies, survivorship has been reported at 90.6%–91.3% for INBONE, 97%–100% for INBONE-II, and 96.6% for both groups combined.[54,55] However, midterm survivorship is less promising in cases of revision (77.8%).[56]

Early-term follow-up studies report consistent improvements in PROs from preoperative states.[8,51,53] A 2015 study comparing INBONE and INBONE-II demonstrated similar significant improvements in AOFAS, SMFA, VAS, and SF-36 score for both groups at 24 months.[53] Hsu and colleagues[57] as well as Wu and colleagues[58] demonstrated similar findings at 3 years for AOFAS, VAS, and SF-36 scores. Significant improvements in AOFAS, VAS, SMFA, and SF-36 have been demonstrated for both primary and revision cases using INBONE and INBONE-2; however, the improvements are less pronounced with revision cohorts. Studies with follow-up from 5 to 8 years show significant improvements in EQ-5D, Manchester-Oxford Foot Questionnaire (MOxFQ), Foot and Ankle Outcome Score (FAOS), VAS, SMFA, AOFAS, SF-36, and patient-reported function.[54,55,59]

INFINITY

The INFINITY Total Ankle System (Wright Medical/Stryker, Memphis, TN, USA) was studied in 20 included articles, with an average follow-up of 37.98 months (16.2–70.37 months). Reports on early survivorship range from 95.3% to 100%.[60] Midterm survivorship has been reported as ranging from 93% to 100%.[61,62]

Short-term follow-up studies demonstrate improvement in PROs using the INFINITY implant. A 2021 multicenter prospective study shows significant improvements in AOS, MOxFQ, and EQ-5D,[60] and a 2018 retrospective cohort study demonstrated significant improvements in FAOS (pain, quality of life, and activities of daily living).[63]

In a midterm follow-up study, Penner and colleagues reported significant improvements in AOS, FFI, SF-36 physical component score (PCS) at 35.4 months.[62] Baumfeld and colleagues reported improvements in VAS and AOFAS at 4 years.[64]

Zimmer trabecular metal

The Zimmer Trabecular Metal Total Ankle (Zimmer Biomet, Warsaw, IN, USA) was included in 17 clinical outcome studies, with an average follow-up of 36.1 months (12–60 months). Short-term survivorship is reported as 93.7%–100%,[8,65] and midterm survivorship ranges from 92.1% to 98%.[66,67]

Early follow-up studies for the Trabecular Metal implant have shown improvements in PROs. A 2021 study showed improved AOFAS, VAS, and SF-12 regardless of valgus deformity.[65] Significant improvements in VAS, FAOS, FFI, and PROMIS (physical functional and pain interference) had been reported in short-term studies. There are a few midterm follow-up studies for the Zimmer implant, showing improvements in AOFAS, VAS, SF-36, EQ-5D, AOS, and SF-12 at 2.5 to 3.5 years and FAOS at 5 years.[66,67]

Criteria 2: Total Ankle Arthroplasty Versus Ankle Arthrodesis

After implant design, TAA versus AA is one of the most published on topics for TAA outcome research studies. This is the focus of Rodriguez-Merchan & Moracia-Ochagavia's "Results of Total Ankle Arthroplasty versus Ankle Arthrodesis, in this issue", so we will keep our discussion brief. We identified a total of 27 clinical outcome studies and 10 systematic review/meta-analyses evaluating TAA against AA. Most short-term studies report similar outcome scores with TAA versus AA. In general, the literature supports similar pain relief with similar or superior pain relief with TAA. The prospective, controlled pivotal trial for the STAR versus AA showed equivalent pain relief with better function after TAA.[68] A prospective multicenter study of 273 patients[69] demonstrated significantly better SMFA and SF-36 scores at 3 years in TAA patients compared with AA. These differences were more pronounced when newer TAA systems were used.[69] Sangeorzan and colleagues[52] reported on a randomized control trial ($n = 414$ TAA vs $n = 103$ AA), demonstrating improvements in both groups for FAAM (Sport and ADL),

SF-36 (PCS and Mental Component Score [MCS]), and VAS, but with significantly greater improvements for TAA in all measurements except pain. A large systematic review from 2022 (n = 898 AA vs n = 1638 TAA) at 3.3 years mean follow-up showed no significant difference in PROMs in 68.7% of patients, with 29.3% of patients having superior PROMs in TAA, compared with only 2% superior PROMs in AA.[42]

Criteria 3: Revision Total Ankle Arthroplasty

We found 11 clinical outcome and one systematic review articles report on PROs in RTAA surgery. A 2023 retrospective study[70] demonstrated improved AOFAS and VAS scores for patients undergoing RTAA at 3 years, with 94.4% survivorship. Behrens reported on their postoperative AOFAS and FFI scores for RTAA, with a survivorship of 77.8% at 4 years after revision.[56] Three studies compared RTAA with conversion AA or tibiotalocalcaneal fusion. In a 2022 systematic review of RTAA, Jennison and colleagues[71] reported that 12/16 outcome scores demonstrated significant improvement with RTAA, compared with only 4/22 outcome score with conversion to AA. A retrospective study comparing RTAA with salvage AA demonstrated better final VAS, MOxFQ, and AOS scores for the RTAA group.[72]

Criteria 4: Coronal Deformity

Ten studies reported on the effect of coronal deformity of TAA outcome scores. Harston and colleagues[59] compared patients with a preoperative coronal deformity ($\geq$10° varus or valgus) to neutral (10° varus–10°) valgus, reporting no difference in outcome scores (AOFAS, SMFA, and SF-36) or revision rates between groups. There were significantly more reoperations in the deformity group, however. Another study compared groups with moderate coronal deformities (5°–15° varus or valgus) to severe coronal deformities (20°–35° varus or valgus). Although all scores improved, they showed no significant intergroup differences for AOS (pain and disability), AOFAS, SF-36 (PCS), and VAS. Survival rates were similar (92.3% severe vs 90.7% moderate) at 74 months.[29]

Studies focusing on valgus deformity report good results despite degree of deformity. Piga and colleagues[65] compared outcomes for neutral (0°–10°) and valgus (>10°) ankles. They reported a significant improvement in AOFAS, VAS, and SF-12 in both groups compared with preoperative measurements. There were no significant difference comparing neutral to valgus deformities outcome scores. Neutral ankles had higher reported survivorship at 2 years (98.6% in neutral vs 94.7% in valgus). Likewise, Demetracopoulos and colleagues[73] reported their results comparing clinical outcomes for moderate (10°–20°) versus severe (>20°) valgus deformities. They noted significant improvements in VAS, SF-36, SMFA, and AOFAS in both groups, without a significant difference between groups. Survivorship was 92% at 42 months overall.[73]

Clinical outcome studies focusing on varus deformities demonstrate improved scores in TAA regardless of varus ankle alignment. Usuelli and colleagues compared neutral (10° valgus–10° varus) to varus ankles (>10° varus alignment).[24] Although AOFAS, VAS, and SF-12 scores improved postoperatively in both groups, there were no differences in scores between groups. Survivorship was 91% varus and 97% in neutral ankles at 3.8 years.[24] In a similar study comparing ankles with varus deformity (>10°) vs (0°–10°), improvements were seen in AOFAS, AOS, and SF-36 scores, but no difference was observed between groups.[74]

Criteria 5: Total Ankle Arthroplasty in Hemophilic Arthropathy of the Ankle

Seven clinical studies and one systematic review investigate PROs in patients with hemophilia associated arthropathy undergoing TAA. These studies often have smaller sample sizes (average sample size $n = 17$, range 9–34 subjects). Barg and colleagues[30] reported significant improvements in VAS and SF-36, with high patient satisfaction. Survivorship was 100% at 5 years. A 2014 study likewise demonstrated significant improvements in AOFAS and VAS, with high satisfaction and 100% survivorship at 3 years. A longer term (115.2 months) follow-up study from 2018 showed SF-36 scores comparable to age-matched norms. Survivorship was 85% at 10 years and 70% at 15 years. A study evaluating TAA versus AA in the hemophilia population reported significantly better results for FFI subscales (disability and activity) for patients undergoing TAA compared with AA.[75]

Criteria 6: Patient Age

Five articles address the effect of age on PROs in patients undergoing TAA. These studies show the efficacy of TAA in improving clinical outcome scores in all age groups. Tenenbaum and colleagues compared elderly (>70 years) to younger (50–60 years) TAA patients.[16] They did not demonstrate any significant differences in postoperative VAS, AOFAS, or SF-36 PCS between groups; however, both groups had significant improvements compared with preoperative measurements. Demetracopoulos and colleagues[76] showed younger patients (<55 years, average age 47.0 years) had significantly greater improvements in postoperative SF-36 (Vitality) compared and AOFAS scores for compared elderly patients (>70 years, average age 76.0 years). Survivorship was 93% in younger patients (<55 years); 94.6% in older (55–70 years); and 94.9% in elderly (>70 years) at 42 months.

Criteria 7: Bilateral Total Ankle Arthroplasty

Six studies investigate the role of bilateral TAA on PROs, with two the investigators investing simultaneous bilateral TAA. Comparing patients who have undergone unilateral TAA versus staged bilateral TAA, Desai and colleagues reported significantly worse preoperative SF-36 scores in the bilateral group. However, both groups showed significantly improved postoperative SF-36 scores, with no significant intergroup differences in the postoperative period.[77] Fletcher and colleagues[78] assessed simultaneous bilateral versus sequential TAA in a 2022 retrospective study ($n = 100$ ankles). The investigators report equivalent significant improvements in VAS, SF-36, and SMFA scores in both groups, with 100% survivorship at 52 months. They conclude that simultaneous bilateral TAA is safe and effective.[78]

TOTAL ANKLE ARTHROPLASTY REGISTRIES

National or international registries are the most complete and effective method of tracking implant longevity and patient outcomes following TAA. National implant registries are an expensive and cumbersome undertaking that requires significant investment of time and resources to initiate and maintain. We are aware of seven active National TAA registries currently tracking implant longevity with very few tracking PROs. The most recent data from each are reviewed below.

United Kingdom (England, Wales, and North Ireland)

The National Joint Registry combines the reports from these countries and is the largest.[79] Data collection compiles primary ankle arthroplasties from January 2010 to December 2021. Through 2022, there were 7849 total ankle arthroplasties included in the registry, and numbers have increased considerably since 2015. The median age was 69 year old and 59.9% were males. No PROs were included in this report.

Longevity
The overall cumulative revision rate at 5 and 10 years was 5.5% and 9.0%, respectively. During this period, 396 cases were revised, with and the most common indication being implant loosening (45.9%) and infection (28.5%), followed by pain, lysis, malalignment, and poly insert wear among others. Revision was higher in patients less than 65 year old. Fixed insert designed implants started to be implemented during 2014 which seemed to improve implant survivorship since its introduction.

Australia

The Australian Orthopedic Association National Joint Replacement Registry is also a large.[80] Their 2022 annual report encompassing 3448 primary TAA (84.4%) and 639 revisions (15.6%) between 2006 and December 2021 had a mean age of 67.1 year old and 61% males. Osteoarthritis (OA) was the most common indication (93.7%), seconded far behind by rheumatoid arthritis (RA, 4.7%). No PROs were disclosed in this report.

Longevity
The cumulative revision rate at 10 years for OA and RA was 15.5% and 14%, respectively. Implant loosening was the most common indication (27.8%), followed by infection (12.3%), lysis (10.4%), and instability (10%), among others. Most common procedure done for revision was poly insert exchange (49.2%), followed by arthrodesis (14.2%). Interestingly, the revision rate has declined since 2015 given a 5-year cumulative percent revision decrease from pre-2015 (10.7%) to post-2015 (5.6%) period. This decrease conincided with increased use of fixed designed inserts. Increasing risk factors for revision were age <55 year old and mobile inserts (11% cumulative percent at 5 years).

New Zealand

The New Zealand Joint Registry 23-year report encompasses 2016 primary total ankle arthroplasties between January 2000 and December 2021.[81] The mean age was 66.7% and 60.7% were males. OA was the most common indication (75.7%), followed by RA (8.2%). Regarding PROs, since 2015, the MOxFQ is used to track outcomes. This was sent to the patients at 6 months post-operatively. Out of 416 responses the mean score was 18.9 (standard deviation, 14.7). This score can range from 0 to 64, 0 being best possible outcome.

Longevity
During this period, the analysis demonstrated an 18-year survival of 78.3%, and 285 cases were revised. The average time to revision was 5 years from index surgery, and the main reasons were implant loosening (36.8%), followed by pain (31.2%) and infection (7.4%), among others.

The Netherlands

The Dutch Arthroplasty Register report from 2022 collects data from surgeries performed from 2014 to 2021.[82] There were 960 primary total ankle arthroplasties. In 2021, the mean age was 69.7 year old and 57% were male. In that year a total of 122 primaries were done, of which 89.3% corresponded to OA. No PROs were disclosed in this report.

Longevity
During this reported period, 214 revisions were done. In 2021, 26 revisions were performed. The most common indications for revisions in 2021 were implant loosening

and cyst formation (53.9%), poly insert wear (30.8%), infection and malalignment (15.4%), and arthrofibrosis, among others. Cumulative revision rate at 5 years was 6.3%.

Sweden

The Swedish Ankle Registry by 2020 reported on 1230 total ankle arthroplasties performed from 1993 to 2016.[83] The mean age was 60 year old, and 60% were females. The most common indication was OA (60%) and RA (24%). No PROs were disclosed in this report.

Longevity
In this period, 22% were revised, being the most common indication implant loosening (45%), followed by poly insert wear (13%), infection (11%), and instability (4%) among others. The cumulative overall survival rate at 5 years was 85%.

Norway

The Norwegian Arthroplasty Register between 1994 and 2021 collected 1368 total ankle arthroplasties.[84] The mean age was 60.3 year old and 53.3% were females. The most common indication for primary arthroplasty was OA (idiopathic and post-traumatic, 57.7%), followed by RA (26.5%). No PROs were disclosed in this report.

Longevity
Regarding revisions, 549 were performed and the most common indications were implant loosening (35.7%), pain (33.1%), poly insert defect (18.5%), malalignment (12.6%), instability (6.2%), and infection (4.7%) among others.

Finland

The Finnish Arthroplasty Register between 1982 and 2006 reporting on those with more than 2 years follow-up and implants used in at least 40 operations had 515 primary total ankle arthroplasties done.[85] The mean age was 55 year old, and 63% were females. The most common indications were RA (49%) and OA (41%). No PROs were disclosed in this report.

Longevity
During this period, 59 (11%) were revised due to implant loosening (39%), instability (39%), or infection (7%) among others. The cumulative overall implant survival rate at 5 years was 83%.

Registries summary

From the collected data found on the seven registries mentioned, the mean age ranged 55 to 69 year old, four had a male predominance ranging 57% to 61%, and OA was the most common indication. The percent of revision is low and varies between registries given different time frames. Based on the provided 5-year cumulative revision rate, it ranged 5.5% to 6.3%, and two of the reports showed a 5-year cumulative implant survival rate above 80%.[83,85] The most common indications encountered for revision were implant loosening, followed by poly insert or pain. In Finland's registry, instability was high as opposed to other countries.[85] Regarding infection rate as indication for revision, the National Joint Registry had the highest rate of all, approximating 30%,[79] whereas on the other registries, it ranged from 15.4% to 4.7%. Interestingly, the Australian Joint Registry noted that there was an improvement in implant longevity from after 2014 due to the introduction and use of fixed implants as reflected by the 5-year cumulative revision rate decline post-2015.[79,80] Only one registry, the New Zealand Joint Registry, collects PROs, and only at 6 months post-op to date.[81]

A ROADMAP FOR THE FUTURE

There are more than 22 different TAA implants with described outcomes in the English literature. The large majority (83%) describe short or intermediate term outcomes (eg, <7 years follow-up). Although early functional results and revision rates are helpful, there is a pressing need to track patient outcomes and implant longevity and to identify risk factors for early revision and suboptimal outcomes. The ideal state would include an inclusive, collaborative American and Canadian North American registry, which mandates secure and careful tracking of implants, implant longevity, PROMs, and patient demographic factors. This should be supported by government and private payors, implant companies, hospitals, and practices. The American Academy of Orthopaedic Surgeons (AAOS) has created a TAA registry to be incorporated into the existing AJRR in 2023.

The second consideration is the PROM used to track outcomes for TAA. In general, the selected metrics should include measures of pain, physical function, and general health. Two of the top 3 metrics listed in **Fig. 1** (AOFAS scale and SF-36) are problematic because AOFAS scales are not validated[3] and SF-36 is a very long survey to use in clinic practice. SMFA is also very long at 46 questions. It can be challenging in clinical practice, particularly in community practice to successfully collect PROMs from patients if there is significant survey burden. The AOS is validated, reliable scale including 18 questions in the domains of pain and disability. The PROMIS measures, conspicuously absent from the current TAA literature, would also be widely supported based on literature trends in foot and ankle[86] and would substantially reduce survey burden. A valuable next step would be a collaborative consensus statement from AOFAS and Canadian Orthopaedic Foot and Ankle Society (COFAS) on appropriate PROMs to be used in TAA outcomes assessment. AOFAS has a current position statement with broad recommendations, but does not specify for specific conditions or procedures.[87]

SUMMARY

TAA is an increasingly common, highly effective treatment for ankle arthritis. As implants continue to improve, our ability to critically assess outcomes, both through PROMs and implant longevity, is vital to optimizing care of this disabling condition. Patient registries which include PROs are difficult to implement and very costly to maintain. However, this would provide the best infrastructure to define and evaluate appropriate patient selection and best practices with regard to postoperative management and activity restrictions. All centers performing these procedures should be encouraged to participate in the AAOS and/or COFAS registry, or critically report their own outcomes. This would arm orthopedic surgeons with the resources and knowledge to continually improve techniques and protocols, and properly educate patients on what they can expect from their TAA.

CLINICS CARE POINTS

- TAA) is an effective treatment for end-stage ankle arthritis.
- There are 22 implants in the market in North America, with increasing evidence of effectiveness.
- There is evidence of good early outcomes in younger patients.
- TAA generally results in similar pain relief with superior function compared with AA.

- There are seven national registries tracking outcomes and longevity of TAAs.
- Only one registry tracks patient-reported outcomes and that only at 6 months post-op.

DISCLOSURE

The authors have nothing relevant to disclose.

REFERENCES

1. Rushing C, Mckenna BJ, Zulauf EA, et al. Intermediate-Term Outcomes of a Third-Generation, 2-Component Total Ankle Prosthesis. Foot Ankle Int 2021; 42(7):935–43.
2. Tucker WA, Barnds BL, Morris BL, et al. Nationwide Analysis of Total Ankle Replacement and Ankle Arthrodesis in Medicare Patients: Trends, Complications, and Cost. Foot Ankle Spec 2022;15(3):201–8.
3. Pinsker E, Daniels TR. AOFAS position statement regarding the future of the AOFAS Clinical Rating Systems. Foot Ankle Int 2011;32(9):841–2.
4. Kitaoka HB, Meeker JE, Phisitkul P, et al. AOFAS Position Statement Regarding Patient-Reported Outcome Measures. Foot Ankle Int 2018;39(12):1389–93.
5. Shah NS UY, Suriel Peguero E, Erwin JT, et al. Laughlin R Outcome Reporting in Total Ankle Arthroplasty: A Systematic Review. J Foot Ankle Surg 2021;60(4): 770–6.
6. Foran IM VE, Bohl DD, Lee S, et al. Quality Assessment of Modern Total Ankle Arthroplasty Clinical Outcomes Research. J Foot Ankle Surg 2022;61(1):7–11.
7. Ahmad SS, Hoos L, Perka C, et al. Follow-up definitions in clinical orthopaedic research: a systematic review. Bone & Joint Open 2021;2(5):344–50.
8. Norvell DC, Ledoux WR, Shofer JB, et al. Effectiveness and Safety of Ankle Arthrodesis Versus Arthroplasty: A Prospective Multicenter Study. J Bone Joint Surg Am 2019;101(16):1485–94.
9. Karantana A, Hobson S, Dhar S. The Scandinavian total ankle replacement: survivorship at 5 and 8 years comparable to other series. Clin Orthop Relat Res 2010;468(4):951–7.
10. Kerkhoff YR, Kosse NM, Metsaars WP, et al. Long-term Functional and Radiographic Outcome of a Mobile Bearing Ankle Prosthesis. Foot Ankle Int 2016; 37(12):1292–302.
11. Palanca A, Mann RA, Mann JA, et al. Scandinavian Total Ankle Replacement: 15-Year Follow-up. Foot Ankle Int 2018;39(2):135–42.
12. Zhao H, Yang Y, Yu G, et al. A systematic review of outcome and failure rate of uncemented Scandinavian total ankle replacement. Int Orthop 2011;35(12): 1751–8.
13. Queen RM, Sparling TL, Butler RJ, et al. Patient-Reported Outcomes, Function, and Gait Mechanics After Fixed and Mobile-Bearing Total Ankle Replacement. J Bone Joint Surg Am 2014;96(12):987–93.
14. Cunningham DJ, DeOrio JK, Nunley JA, et al. The Effect of Patient Characteristics on 1 to 2-Year and Minimum 5-Year Outcomes After Total Ankle Arthroplasty. J Bone Joint Surg Am 2019;101(3):199–208.
15. Scott DJ, Kane J, Ford S, et al. Correlation of Patient-Reported Outcomes With Physical Function After Total Ankle Arthroplasty. Foot Ankle Int 2021;42(5): 646–53.

16. Tenenbaum S, Bariteau J, Coleman S, et al. Functional and clinical outcomes of total ankle arthroplasty in elderly compared to younger patients. Foot Ankle Surg 2017;23(2):102–7.
17. Daniels TR, Mayich DJ, Penner MJ. Intermediate to Long-Term Outcomes of Total Ankle Replacement with the Scandinavian Total Ankle Replacement (STAR). J Bone Joint Surg Am 2015;97(11):895–903.
18. Nunley JA, Caputo AM, Easley ME, et al. Intermediate to long-term outcomes of the STAR Total Ankle Replacement: the patient perspective. J Bone Joint Surg Am 2012;94(1):43–8.
19. Loewy EM, Sanders TH, Walling AK. Intermediate-term Experience With the STAR Total Ankle in the United States. Foot Ankle Int 2019;40(3):268–75.
20. Mann JA, Mann RA, Horton E. STAR ankle: long-term results. Foot Ankle Int 2011; 32(5):S473–84.
21. Jastifer JR, Coughlin MJ. Long-term follow-up of mobile bearing total ankle arthroplasty in the United States. Foot Ankle Int 2015;36(2):143–50.
22. Koivu H, Kohonen I, Mattila K, et al. Long-term Results of Scandinavian Total Ankle Replacement. Foot Ankle Int 2017;38(7):723–31.
23. Raglan M, Machin JT, Cro S, et al. Total ankle replacement : comparison of the outcomes of STAR and Mobility. Acta Orthop Belg 2020;86(1):109–14.
24. Usuelli FG, Di Silvestri CA, D'Ambrosi R, et al. Total ankle replacement: is preoperative varus deformity a predictor of poor survival rate and clinical and radiological outcomes? Int Orthop 2019;43(1):243–9.
25. Lee KB, Kim MS, Park KS, et al. Effect of anterior translation of the talus on outcomes of three-component total ankle arthroplasty. BMC Musculoskelet Disord 2013;14:260.
26. Strauss AC, Goldmann G, Wessling M, et al. Total ankle replacement in patients with haemophilia and virus infections–a safe alternative to ankle arthrodesis? Haemophilia 2014;20(5):702–8.
27. Lefrancois T, Younger A, Wing K, et al. A Prospective Study of Four Total Ankle Arthroplasty Implants by Non-Designer Investigators. J Bone Joint Surg Am 2017;99(4):342–8.
28. Van Haecke A, Semay B, Fessy MH, et al. 97 HINTEGRA ankle prostheses: Results and survival at more than 5 years' follow-up. Foot Ankle Surg 2022;28(8):1241–7.
29. Lee GW, Lee KB. Outcomes of Total Ankle Arthroplasty in Ankles with >20 degrees of Coronal Plane Deformity. J Bone Joint Surg Am 2019;101(24):2203–11.
30. Barg A, Elsner A, Hefti D, et al. Total ankle arthroplasty in patients with hereditary hemochromatosis. Clin Orthop Relat Res 2011;469(5):1427–35.
31. Clifton LJ, Kingman A, Rushton PRP, et al. The Hintegra total ankle replacement: survivorship, failure modes and patient reported outcomes in seventy consecutive cases with a minimum five year follow-up. Int Orthop 2021;45(9):2331–6.
32. Mussawy H, Kehrer M, Strahl A, et al. Clinical and patient reported outcome in total ankle replacement compared to ankle fusion in end-stage haemophilic arthropathy. Haemophilia 2021;27(6):e739–46.
33. Yoon YK, Park KH, Park JH, et al. Long-Term Clinical Outcomes and Implant Survivorship of 151 Total Ankle Arthroplasties Using the HINTEGRA Prosthesis: A Minimum 10-Year Follow-up. J Bone Joint Surg Am 2022;104(16):1483–91.
34. Kvarda P, Peterhans US, Susdorf R, et al. Long-Term Survival of HINTEGRA Total Ankle Replacement in 683 Patients: A Concise 20-Year Follow-up of a Previous Report. J Bone Joint Surg Am 2022;104(10):881–8.

35. Kim TY, Lee HW, Jeong BO. Influence of Depressive Symptoms on the Clinical Outcomes of Total Ankle Arthroplasty. J Foot Ankle Surg 2020;59(1):59–63.

36. McGurk KM, Scott DJ, Hoch C, et al. Sex Differences in Patient-Reported Outcomes and Range of Motion After Total Ankle Arthroplasty. Foot Ankle Spec 2023. https://doi.org/10.1177/19386400231168737. 19386400231168737.

37. Barg A, Knupp M, Hintermann B. Simultaneous bilateral versus unilateral total ankle replacement: a patient-based comparison of pain relief, quality of life and functional outcome. J Bone Joint Surg Br 2010;92(12):1659–63.

38. Joo SD, Lee KB. Comparison of the outcome of total ankle arthroplasty for osteoarthritis with moderate and severe varus malalignment and that with neutral alignment. Bone Joint Lett J 2017;99-B(10):1335–42.

39. Conlin C, Khan RM, Wilson I, et al. Living With Both a Total Ankle Replacement and an Ankle Fusion: A Qualitative Study From the Patients' Perspective. Foot Ankle Int 2021;42(9):1153–61.

40. Sung KS, Ahn J, Lee KH, et al. Short-term results of total ankle arthroplasty for end-stage ankle arthritis with severe varus deformity. Foot Ankle Int 2014;35(3):225–31.

41. Bai LB, Lee KB, Song EK, et al. Total ankle arthroplasty outcome comparison for post-traumatic and primary osteoarthritis. Foot Ankle Int 2010;31(12):1048–56.

42. Gajebasia S, Jennison T, Blackstone J, et al. Patient reported outcome measures in ankle replacement versus ankle arthrodesis - A systematic review. Foot 2022;51:101874.

43. Veljkovic AN, Daniels TR, Glazebrook MA, et al. Outcomes of Total Ankle Replacement, Arthroscopic Ankle Arthrodesis, and Open Ankle Arthrodesis for Isolated Non-Deformed End-Stage Ankle Arthritis. J Bone Joint Surg Am 2019;101(17):1523–9.

44. Hendy BA, McDonald EL, Nicholson K, et al. Improvement of Outcomes During the First Two Years Following Total Ankle Arthroplasty. J Bone Joint Surg Am 2018;100(17):1473–81.

45. Gross CE, Green CL, DeOrio JK, et al. Impact of Diabetes on Outcome of Total Ankle Replacement. Foot Ankle Int 2015;36(10):1144–9.

46. Day J, Kim J, O'Malley MJ, et al. Radiographic and Clinical Outcomes of the Salto Talaris Total Ankle Arthroplasty. Foot Ankle Int 2020;41(12):1519–28.

47. Vesely BD, King MA, Scott AT. Intermediate to Long-Term Follow-up of the Salto Talaris Fixed-Bearing Total Ankle Prosthesis. Foot Ankle Spec 2023;16(3):267–72.

48. McConnell EP, Queen RM. Correlation of Physical Performance and Patient-Reported Outcomes Following Total Ankle Arthroplasty. Foot Ankle Int 2017;38(2):115–23.

49. Steele JR, Cunningham DJ, Green CL, et al. Patient Characteristics of Possible Responders and Nonresponders to Total Ankle Arthroplasty. Foot Ankle Int 2020;41(8):893–900.

50. Akoh CC, Fletcher AN, Chen J, et al. Economic Analysis and Clinical Outcomes of Short-Stay Versus Inpatient Total Ankle Replacement Surgery. Foot Ankle Int 2021;42(1):96–106.

51. Coetzee JC, Petersen D, Stone RM. Comparison of Three Total Ankle Replacement Systems Done at a Single Facility. Foot Ankle Spec 2017;10(1):20–5.

52. Sangeorzan BJ, Ledoux WR, Shofer JB, et al. Comparing 4-Year Changes in Patient-Reported Outcomes Following Ankle Arthroplasty and Arthrodesis. J Bone Joint Surg Am 2021;103(10):869–78.

53. Lewis JS Jr, Green CL, Adams SB, et al. Comparison of First- and Second-Generation Fixed-Bearing Total Ankle Arthroplasty Using a Modular Intramedullary Tibial Component. Foot Ankle Int 2015;36(8):881–90.

54. Gagne OJ, Day J, Kim J, et al. Midterm Survivorship of the INBONE II Total Ankle Arthroplasty. Foot Ankle Int 2022;43(5):628–36.

55. Jamjoom BA, Siddiqui BM, Salem H, et al. Clinical and Radiographic Outcomes of Revision Total Ankle Arthroplasty Using the INBONE II Prosthesis. J Bone Joint Surg Am 2022;104(17):1554–62.

56. Behrens SB, Irwin TA, Bemenderfer TB, et al. Clinical and Radiographic Outcomes of Revision Total Ankle Arthroplasty Using an Intramedullary-Referencing Implant. Foot Ankle Int 2020;41(12):1510–8.

57. Hsu AH. Early Clinical and Radiographic Outcomes of Intramedullary-Fixation Total Ankle Arthroplasty. J Bone Joint Surg Am 2015;97(3):194–200.

58. Wu Y, Y H, Guo X, et al. Total ankle replacement with INBONE-II prosthesis: A short-to- medium-term follow-up study in China. China Med J 2022;135(12):1459–65.

59. Harston A LA, Adams SB Jr, DeOrio JK, et al. Midterm outcomes of a fixed-bearing total ankle arthroplasty with deformity analysis. Foot Ankle Int 2017;38(12):1295–300.

60. Townshend DN, Bing AJF, Clough TM, et al. Early experience and patient-reported outcomes of 503 INFINITY total ankle arthroplasties. Bone Joint J 2021;103:1270–6.

61. Pierce Ebaugh M, Alford T, Kutzarov K, et al. Patient-Reported Outcomes of Primary Total Ankle Arthroplasty in Patients Aged <50 Years. Foot Ankle Orthop 2022;7(1). https://doi.org/10.1177/24730114221082601. 24730114221082601.

62. Penner M, Wing K, Bemenderfer T, et al. The Infinity Total Ankle System: Early Clinical Results With 2- to 4-Year Follow-up. Foot Ankle Spec 2019;12(2):159–66.

63. Saito GH, Sanders AE, de Cesar Netto C, et al. Short-term complications, reoperations, and radiographic outcomes of a new fixed-bearing total ankle arthroplasty. Foot Ankle Int 2018;39(7):787–94.

64. Baumfeld D, Baumfeld T, Fernandes Rezende R, et al. Infinity Ankle Arthroplasty Early Latin-America Experience and Patient Outcomes. Foot Ankle Spec 2023;16(3):226–32.

65. Piga C MC, D'Ambrosi R, Romano F, et al. Total Ankle Arthroplasty With Valgus Deformity. Foot Ankle Int 2021;42(7):867–76.

66. Kim J, Gagne OJ, Rajan L, et al. Clinical outcomes of the lateral trabecular metal total ankle replacement at a 5-year minimum follow-up. Foot Ankle Spec 2023;16(3):288–99.

67. Mosca M, Vocale E, Maitan N, et al. Clinical-radiological outcomes and complications after total ankle replacement through a lateral transfibular approach: a retrospective evaluation at a mid-term follow-up. Int Orthop 2021;45(2):437–43.

68. Saltzman CL, Mann RA, Ahrens JE, et al. Prospective controlled trial of STAR total ankle replacement versus ankle fusion: initial results. Foot Ankle Int 2009;30(7):579–96.

69. Benich MR, Ledoux WR, Orendurff MS, et al. Comparison of Treatment Outcomes of Arthrodesis and Two Generations of Ankle Replacement Implants. J Bone Joint Surg Am 2017;99(21):1792–800.

70. Kvarda P, Toth L, Horn-Lang T, et al. How Does a Novel In Situ Fixed-bearing Implant Design Perform in Revision Ankle Arthroplasty in the Short Term? A Survival, Clinical, and Radiologic Analysis. Clin Orthop Relat Res 2023;481(7):1360–70.

71. Jennison T, Spolton-Dean C, Rottenburg H, et al. The outcomes of revision surgery for a failed ankle arthroplasty : a systematic review and meta-analysis. Bone Jt Open 2022;3(7):596–606.
72. Egglestone A, Kakwani R, Aradhyula M, et al. Outcomes of revision surgery for failed total ankle replacement: revision arthroplasty versus arthrodesis. Int Orthop 2020;44(12):2727–34.
73. Demetracopoulos CA CE, Adams SB Jr, DeOrio JK, et al. Outcomes of Total Ankle Arthroplasty in Moderate and Severe Valgus Deformity. Foot Ankle Spec 2019; 12(3):238–45.
74. Trajkovski T PE, Cadden A, Daniels T, et al. Outcomes of ankle arthroplasty with preoperative coronal-plane varus deformity of 10° or greater. J Bone Joint Surg Am 2013;95(15):1382–8.
75. Ahn J, Yoo MC, Seo J, et al. Comparison of Total Ankle Arthroplasty and Ankle Arthrodesis in End-Stage Hemophilic Arthropathy. Foot Ankle Int 2020;41(8):937–44.
76. Demetracopoulos CA, Adams SB, Queen RM, et al. Effect of Age on Outcomes in Total Ankle Arthroplasty. Foot Ankle Int 2015;36(8):871–80.
77. Desai SJ, Glazebrook M, Penner MJ, et al. Quality of Life in Bilateral Vs. Unilateral End-Stage Ankle Arthritis and Outcomes of Bilateral Vs. Unilateral Total Ankle Replacement. J Bone Joint Surg Am 2017;99(2):133–40.
78. Fletcher AN, Johnson LG, Easley ME, et al. Clinical Outcomes and Complications of Simultaneous or Sequential Bilateral Total Ankle Arthroplasty: A Single-Center Comparative Cohort Study. J Bone Joint Surg Am 2022;104(19):1712–21.
79. The National Joint Registry. 19th Annual Report. 2022: 1-374. cited 2023 5/20 ; Available from: https://reports.njrcentre.org.uk/AR-Executive-Summary.
80. Australian Orthopaedic Association National Joint Replacement Registry. Demographics and Outcomes of Ankle Arthroplasty: Supplementary Report. In: Hip, knee & shoulder arthroplasty: 2022 annual report. Adelaide: AOA; 2022. p. 1–30, cited 2023 5/15; Available at: https://aoanjrr.sahmri.com/annual-reports-2022/supplementary.
81. The New Zealand Joint Registry. Twenty-Three Year Report January 1999 to December 2021. 2023: 1-236 cited 2023 5/18; Available at: https://www.nzoa.org.nz/nzoa-joint-registry.
82. Dutch Arthroplasty Register. LROI Report. 2022: 1-214 cited 2023 5/22; Available at: http://www.lroi-rapportage.nl/.
83. Undén A, Jehpsson L, Kamrad I, et al. Better implant survival with modern ankle prosthetic designs: 1,226 total ankle prostheses followed for up to 20 years in the Swedish Ankle Registry. Acta Orthop 2020;91(2):191–6.
84. Haukeland University Hospital. Norwegian National Advisory Unit on Arthroplasty and Hip Fractures Report. 2022: 1-376 cited 2023 5/30; Available at: https://helse-bergen.no/seksjon/Nasjonal_kompetansetjeneste_leddproteser_hoftebrudd/Share%20point%20Documents/Rapport/Report%202022%20english.pdf.
85. Skyttä ET, Koivu H, Eskelinen A, et al. Total ankle replacement: a population-based study of 515 cases from the Finnish Arthroplasty Register. Acta Orthop 2010;81(1):114–8.
86. Czerwonka N, Desai SS, Arciero E, et al. Contemporary Review: An Overview of the Utility of Patient-Reported Outcome Measurement Information System (PROMIS) in Foot and Ankle Surgery. Foot Ankle Int 2023;44(6):554–64.
87. AOFAS. POSTION STATEMENT Patient-Reported Outcomes Measures 2023 cited 2023 8/26/2023; Available from: https://www.aofas.org/docs/default-source/research-and-policy/position-statements/patient-reported-outcomes-measures-position-statement.pdf?sfvrsn=c866ee8e_4.

Results of Total Ankle Arthroplasty Versus Ankle Arthrodesis

Emerito Carlos Rodriguez-Merchan, MD, PhD*,
Inmaculada Moracia-Ochagavia, MD

KEYWORDS

- Ankle • Total ankle arthroplasty • Ankle arthrodesis • Results

KEY POINTS

- No differences have been found between total ankle arthroplasty (TAA) and ankle arthrodesis (AA) with respect to patient-reported outcome measures.
- Two-year complication rates were higher after AA (27%) than after TAA (16%). Infection rates were similar (4%).
- The published revision rate after AA is 16% versus 11% after TAA.
- Given the insufficient level of evidence in recent publications, their conclusions are not definitive in terms of which operation is more suitable in advanced ankle osteoarthritis. Therefore, more and better designed studies are required.

INTRODUCTION

When conservative treatment (analgesics, anti-inflammatory drugs, canes, unloading orthoses), alone or in combination with intraarticular injections of corticosteroids or hyaluronic acid and joint-preserving surgical treatment (arthroscopic debridement, realignment osteotomy, distraction arthroplasty), fails in patients with painful, advanced-stage ankle osteoarthritis (OA), there are 2 surgical options that do not preserve the joint: tibiotalar (TT) arthrodesis (ankle arthrodesis [AA]) or total ankle arthroplasty (TAA). Traditionally, AA has been advised, albeit with a nonunion rate of approximately 10% (requiring reoperation) and a high prevalence of eventual OA in adjacent joints.[1]

TAA was developed to preserve ankle mobility and prevent OA in the adjacent joints. However, as with all types of arthroplasty, TAA experiences wear with use, prompting the majority of surgeons to favor TAA in older, lower demand patients and favoring AA

Department of Orthopedic Surgery, La Paz University Hospital-IdiPaz, Paseo de la Castellana 261, 28046-Madrid, Spain
* Corresponding author. Department of Orthoxpedic Surgery, La Paz University Hospital-IdiPaz, Paseo de la Castellana 261, Madrid 28046, Spain.
E-mail address: ecrmerchan@hotmail.com

Foot Ankle Clin N Am 29 (2024) 27–52
https://doi.org/10.1016/j.fcl.2023.08.010
1083-7515/24/© 2023 Elsevier Inc. All rights reserved.

in younger patients with higher demand. More recently, improvements in TAA design, instrumentation, and surgical technique have expanded the indications for TAA to use in younger patients. The challenge of which intervention, AA or TAA, offers better results remains. In 2022, we published a systematic review comparing TAAs and AAs performed from 2006 to 2020, using patient-reported outcome measures (PROMs), reoperation rates, revision rates, and complications as endpoints. We found no clear evidence of superiority of TAA over AA at 2-year follow-up. However, we noted that such a conclusion may be debatable in patients with diabetes, post-traumatic OA, and hindfoot/midfoot stiffness.[2]

In the current article, we review and compare results of all relevant TAA and AA studies published in PubMed in 2022. We aim to determine whether either procedure showed superiority over the other in terms of PROMs and reoperation, revision, and complication rates. We discuss recent results from the relevant literature on AA, followed by those on TAA, and finally those from studies comparing the 2 techniques.

ANKLE ARTHRODESIS RESULTS IN THE YEAR 2022

Using "ankle arthrodesis" as keyword, 25 PubMed-referenced articles were published in 2022 (up to November 9, 2022), of which 16 directly related to surgical intervention and were included in our analysis. The results of this literature search are summarized in **Table 1**.[3–18]

In all 16 case series in patients with end-stage ankle arthritis, after AA, the average American Orthopaedic Foot and Ankle Score (AOFAS), Visual Analog Scale (VAS), Short Form-12 (SF-12), and Ankle Osteoarthritis Scale (AOS), the PROMs improved. **Fig. 1** shows a case of AA with a good result. In Morasiewicz and colleagues' comparison of Ilizarov external fixation and cannulated screws for AA, the AOFAS scores were similar.[7] Abuhantash and colleagues reported better AOS and Ankle Arthritis scores for arthroscopic AA versus open AA.[14] The investigation by Liu and colleagues, which compared AA performed with concomitant mosaic bone autograft transplantation in patients with or without large talar cysts, the AOFAS proved better in cases without large talar cysts.[17]

Complications were also noted in this group of 16 articles on AA. Fadhel and colleagues reported a revision rate of 11.3%, and theirs was the only study to cite this parameter.[13] The same authors cited a reoperation rate of 12.4% using tibiotalocalcaneal (TTC) arthrodesis with a short retrograde transplantar intramedullary nailing.[13] Of note is the high complication rate reported (19%), with a union rate of 94.5%. Wong and colleagues reported that nonunion had a 3-year probability of 16%, and infection, a 3-year probability of 6%.[10] Mehdi and colleagues' comparison of primary AA and AA after failed TAA (using a posterior iliac crest allograft for filling bone defects) demonstrated similar AOFAS results and similar complication (12% in both groups) and nonunion (6% in both groups) rates.[18] **Fig. 2** shows a failed AA that had to be converted to a TAA, the final result of which was satisfactory.

TOTAL ANKLE ARTHROPLASTY RESULTS IN THE YEAR 2022

Using "total ankle arthroplasty" as keyword, 350 PubMed articles were identified for 2022 (up to November 9, 2022), of which 23 directly related to surgical intervention and were included in our analysis. The results of this literature search are summarized in **Table 2**.[19–41]

In all 23 case series in patients with end-stage ankle arthritis, after TAA, the average AOFAS, VAS, SF-12, and AOS, the PROMs scores improved. **Fig. 3** shows a case of TAA for rheumatoid arthritis with a good result. Revision rates ranged from 10% to

Table 1
Results of ankle arthrodesis in patients with ankle osteoarthritis in recent literature (year 2022)

Authors [Reference]	Type of Study	LoE	N	PROMs	Revision Rate	Reoperation Rate	Complication Rate	Conclusions
Stoltny et al,[3] 2022	Case series	NA	19	Significant improvement of AOFAS, SF-12, and VAS scores	NA	NA	NA	TTCA using an IM nail improved QoL, alleviated pain, and enabled most individuals to move independently
Patel et al,[4] 2022	SR and MA	NA	624	NA	NA	NA	High nonunion rates	TTCA was an effective salvage procedure prior peripheral neuropathic diseases had strong evidence for failure to develop union.
van den Heuvel et al,[5] 2022	Case series: comparative study: 14 plates, 20 screws, 8 IM nails	NA	42	NA	NA	NA	21% (3% nonunion)	Good clinical outcomes for various techniques of fixation in open AA were achieved. The plate-fixation group demonstrated significantly higher infections when compared with screw and IM nail fixation

(continued on next page)

Table 1
(continued)

Authors [Reference]	Type of Study	LoE	N	PROMs	Revision Rate	Reoperation Rate	Complication Rate	Conclusions
Martinelli et al,[6] 2022	Case series: comparative study	NA	44	NA	NA	NA	Union rate was higher (90.5% vs 65.2%) and complication rate was lower (14.3% vs 47.8%) in the arthroscopic group.	Individuals who experienced arthroscopic AA reported better pain control, with greater improvements in VAS for pain scores.
Morasiewicz et al,[7] 2023	Case series: 21 Ilizarov external fixators vs 26 cannulated screws	NA	47	Similar AOFAS scores	NA	NA	NA	AA yielded good subjective and objective results of treatment in both groups, although slightly better results in the Ilizarov group were observed.
Shah et al,[8] 2022	Case series: 46 open AA vs 41 arthroscopic AA (high risk individuals)	III	87	NA	NA	NA	The nonunion rate was 11% in the open and 12% in the arthroscopic group.	Nonunion rates were comparable between open AA and arthroscopic AA in high-risk individuals.
Li et al,[9] 2022	Case series: Ilizarov apparatus (varus ankle OA)	NA	63	AOFAS, VAS improved	NA	NA	Three superficial pin-tract infections solved with local dressing and antibiotic treatment. Two cases of subtalar OA solved with conservative treatment.	AA using the Ilizarov technique was efficient in treating end-stage varus ankle OA.

Study	Study design	Level of evidence	N				Results	Conclusions
Wong et al,[10] 2022	Database study	III	2463	NA	NA	NA	Nonunion occurred in 11% of individuals within 1 y of AA and 16% of individuals within 3 y. Infection occurred in 3.9% of individuals within 1 y of AA and in 6.2% of individuals within 3 y.	The risk of nonunion after AA was highest in obese individuals; the risk of infection after AA was highest in individuals with diabetes or with an elevated Elixhauser Comorbidity Index score.
Coye et al[11]	SR and MA	NA	5793	NA	NA	NA	Nonunion rate was 8% on average. The highest rate of nonunion occurred during TTCA with 27%	The reported nonunion rates were lower than previously published.
Chalak et al,[12] 2022	Case series: internal fixation of ankle fractures complicated by infection, posttraumatic infected ankle arthritis, and osteomyelitis	NA	20	According to the ASAMI criteria, 17 patients had excellent bone scores and 18 patients had good functional scores.	NA	NA	4 individuals had pin-tract infection and 1 had wire breakage of the forefoot ring.	The Ilizarov fixator for AA rendered an excellent way for solid bone fusion, infection elimination, and early weight-bearing.
Fadhel et al,[13] 2022	SR (TTCA with retrograde TIMN)	NA	229	NA	3%	12% rate (with short nail)	19%	The utilization of a short nail led to a higher rate of peri implant complication (2%) and a higher rate of revision (12%).

(continued on next page)

Table 1
(continued)

Authors [Reference]	Type of Study	LoE	N	PROMs	Revision Rate	Reoperation Rate	Complication Rate	Conclusions
Abuhantash et al,[14] 2022	Case series: comparison between 128 open AAs and 223 arthroscopic AAs	III	351	The AOS score and AAS were better in the arthroscopic AA group	NA	NA	Malunion or nonunion was similar in both groups (6% in the arthroscopic AA group, compared with 4% in the open AA group). Deep infection and wound complications did not happen in the arthroscopic AA group but happened in 4% of the individuals in the open AA group.	Arthroscopic AA had a similar revision rate but lower infection rate than open AA.
Reinke et al,[15] 2022	Case series: 10 acute or chronic infections with joint destruction, 9 with posttraumatic necrosis of the talus or Charcot arthropathy. TTCA was performed with Ilizarov apparatus	NA	19	Modified AOFAS score improved.	NA	NA	One individual had partial consolidation, and 4 individuals presented nonunion.	TTCA using the Ilizarov apparatus was performed in difficult cases. The healing rates were below the rates reported in the literature for TTCA in comparable clinical circumstances.

Cifaldi et al,[16] 2022	SR and MA (TTCA using a structural allograft and retrograde IM nail or a plate)	NA	175 (large osseous defects)	NA	NA	27%; 33% nonunion rate	TTCA with use of a structural allograft was a viable treatment alternative for limb salvage for complex hindfoot and ankle pathology involving large osseous defects.
Liu et al,[17] 2022	Case series: comparison between 10 cases of ankle OA with large talar cysts (group 1) vs 10 cases without large talar cysts (group 2). AA was combined with a concomitant procedure of mosaic bone autograft transplantation	NA	20	The AOFAS scores of group 2 were lower than those of group 1	The incidence of complication (10%) in group 1 was significantly lower than that in group 2 (40%).	The use of TTCA combined with mosaic bone autograft transfer was an effective alternative for the treatment of end-stage ankle OA with large talar cysts.

(continued on next page)

Table 1
(continued)

Authors [Reference]	Type of Study	LoE	N	PROMs	Revision Rate	Reoperation Rate	Complication Rate	Conclusions
Mehdi et al,[18] 2022	Case series: comparison between 16 rTTAs performed for failed arthroplasties that caused pain and a functional disability with 16 primary TTAs performed for painful ankle OA	IV	32	AOFAS scores were similar at the last follow-up.	NA	NA	Both groups had similar nonunion (6%) and complication rates (12%)	The rTTA technique using a posterior iliac crest allograft for filling bone defects yielded good functional results.

Abbreviations: AA, ankle arthrodesis; AAS, ankle arthritis score; AOFAS, American Orthopaedic Foot and Ankle Score; AOS, Ankle Osteoarthritis Scale; ASAMI, Association for the Study and Application of the Method of Ilizarov; IM, intramedullary; LoE, level of evidence; MA, meta-analysis; N, number of patients; NA, not available; OA, ankle osteoarthritis; PROMs, patient-reported outcome measures; QoL, Quality of life; rTTA, revision tibiotalar arthrodesis; SF-12, Short form-12; SR, systematic review; TIMN, transplantar intramedullary nailing; TTA, tibiotalar arthrodesis; TTCA, tibio-talo-calcaneal arthrodesis; VAS, Visual Analog Scale.

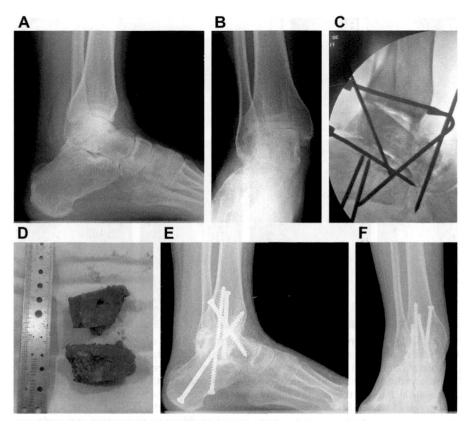

Fig. 1. (*A-F*) Patient with necrosis of the talar body after fracture. She developed tibiotalar and subtalar OA causing pain and disability: (*A*) Lateral radiograph of right ankle showing increased bone density and sclerosis of the talar body compatible with avascular necrosis, nonunion of the talar body fracture, and tibiotalar and subtalar OA; (*B*) AP weight-bearing image of right ankle showing severe joint impingement of the tibiotalar joint; (*C*) Intraoperative lateral radiograph of the right ankle showing provisional ankle fixation for arthrodesis. It should be noted that the necrotic talar body was completely resected and replaced with a tricortical posterior iliac crest graft; (*D*) Image of the tricortical double posterior iliac crest graft; (*E*) Lateral radiograph of the right ankle showing the consolidated arthrodesis in the tibiotalar and subtalar joints; (*F*) AP image of the right ankle showing correct alignment of the ankle and complete consolidation. The patient was satisfied with the result. AP, anteroposterior; OA, osteoarthritis.

28%. Reoperation rates ranged from 8% to 40%. Complication rates ranged from 13% to 23% [See **Table 2**]. **Fig. 4** shows a TAA with talar component loosening, prompting revision TAA, which ultimately resulted in a satisfactory outcome.

COMPARATIVE STUDIES OF ANKLE ARTHRODESIS VERSUS TOTAL ANKLE ARTHROPLASTY IN THE YEARS 2021 AND 2022

To compare studies and outcomes of the 2 surgical techniques, a PubMed search was performed on November 9, 2022, for the years 2021 and 2022; the following keywords were used: total ankle arthroplasty versus ankle arthrodesis (27 results); total ankle replacement versus ankle arthrodesis (24 results); total ankle replacement versus

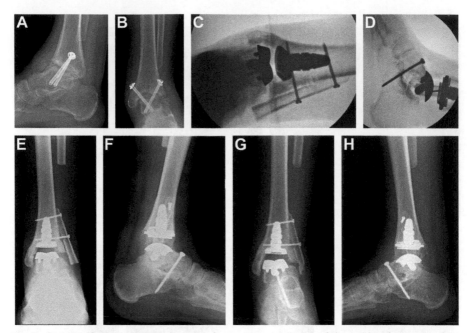

Fig. 2. (*A-H*) Patient who underwent AA for posttraumatic OA of the ankle. The result of the arthrodesis was not good, presenting nonunion of the tibiotalar joint and disabling pain: (*A*) Lateral radiograph of the ankle showing nonunion of previous attempted arthrodesis by osteosynthesis with 2 compression screws; (*B*) AP image of the ankle showing an absence of the distal third of the fibula that was resected during the arthrodesis surgery; (*C*) AP radiograph of the ankle. Surgery was performed to convert the failed AA into a TAA with an intramedullary tibial stem. In the same operation, fibula reconstruction was performed with flipping of the distal end of the fibula; (*D*) Lateral radiograph of the ankle showing good alignment of the prosthetic components. Subtalar joint arthrodesis was also performed; (*E*) AP ankle image 2 months after surgery; (*F*) Lateral ankle radiograph 2 months after surgery; (*G*) AP ankle image 2 years after implantation of the TAA. Thinning of the tip of the reconstructed fibula was performed; (*H*) Lateral ankle radiograph 2 years after surgery. The subtalar joint had consolidated and the prosthetic components remained well aligned with no signs of loosening or mobilization. AA, ankle arthrodesis; AP, anteroposterior; OA, osteoarthritis; TAA, total ankle arthroplasty.

ankle fusion (11 results); and total ankle arthroplasty versus ankle fusion (18 results). Several studies proved to be from the same patient cohorts. We identified 15 articles that qualified for our analysis.

Comparison of Outcomes Between Total Ankle Arthroplasty and Ankle Arthrodesis for Ankle Osteoarthritis Using Real-World Data

In a level III of evidence study, Randsborg and colleagues used state claims data from New York between October 2015 and December 2018 and from California between October 2015 and December 2017.[42] The primary outcome measure was revision. Secondary parameters were in-hospital complications and below-knee amputation. A total of 1477 (50%) TAAs and 1468 (50%) AAs were analyzed. Individuals who had experienced a TAA had fewer comorbidities than those operated on with AA. The TAA group had a lower risk of revision (5% vs 9%), in-hospital complications

Table 2
Results of total ankle arthroplasty in patients with ankle osteoarthritis in recent literature (year 2022)

Authors [Reference]	Type of Study	LoE	N	PROMs	Revision Rate	Reoperation Rate	Complication Rate	Conclusions
Loveday et al,[19] 2022	Case series: 108 Mobility, 19 Zenith, 30 Infinity	NA	157	NA	9.6% at a mean 4 y	NA	Aseptic loosening was the most common reason for revision	Overall survivorship analysis for 5, 10, and 15 y was respectively 92.4%, 89.3%, and 86.6%. TAA provided good functional outcomes and medium term implant survivorship.
Hauer et al,[20] 2022	SR of level III studies	III	5806	NA	12.6% at 7 y	NA	NA	Revision rates of clinical studies and arthroplasty registers were comparable.
Maccario et al,[21] 2022	Case series: transfibular TAA	NA	86	AOFAS, SF-12 and VAS improved	At 5-y FU, 97.7% of implants were free from revision or removal with 84 implants at risk.	NA	2% failures for aseptic loosening	Transfibular TAA was safe and effective with a high survival rate at mid-term FU.
Best et al,[22] 2022	Database analysis	III	294	NA	NA	NA	SSI was the most frequent complication. Diabetes and smoking were associated with greater odds of complications.	TAA had a low complication rate, with SSI being the most common complication. Individuals with diabetes have greater odds of

(continued on next page)

Table 2
(continued)

Authors [Reference]	Type of Study	LoE	N	PROMs	Revision Rate	Reoperation Rate	Complication Rate	Conclusions
								poor results after TAA than individuals without diabetes. Obesity was not associated with poor outcomes after TAA.
Dagneaux et al,[23] 2022	Database analysis	IV	4748	NA	Revisions were required in 817 individuals (17%), including 734 with metal component revision and 83 with revision due to deep infection.	NA	83 deep infections (requiring revision)	The 1-y, 2-y, 5-y, and 10-y survivorship free of metal component revision was 95%, 90%, 84%, and 78%.
Gagne et al,[24] 2022	Case series: INBONE II TAA	IV	51 ankles (46 patients)	All FAOS domain scores improved between preoperative and final FU.		The rate of reoperation was 7.8% (4 patients)	2 individuals required irrigation and debridement for infection, 1 individual experienced a medializing calcaneal osteotomy, 1 individual had open gutter debridement, and 1 individual required a revision of a subsided talar component at 3.2 y after index surgery.	PROMs improved after INBONE II TAA. These patients also had a high rate of survivorship.

Author	Description									
Mo and Ficke[25]	Review article on the most cited TAA design in the literature	V	NA	NA	NA	NA	NA	NA	NA	The most cited TAA design was STAR (15), followed by Agility (7), Buechel-Pappas (5), and Salto (4).
Consul et al,[26] 2022	Case series: individuals younger than 55 y	NA	51	NA	NA	NA	13	13% major complications, 15% minor complications	NA	TAA was a viable treatment alternative for individuals younger than 55 y
Shah et al,[27] 2022	National Inpatient Sample (USA) query (2005–2017)	NA	NA	NA	NA	NA	NA	NA	NA	The prevalence of both TAAs and rTAAs was projected to significantly increase over the next 10 y.
Hermus et al,[28] 2022	SR and MA	NA	16,964 TAAs	NA	NA	NA	NA	Complications with highest reported pooled incidence were intraoperative fracture 0.06 and impingement 0.06, respectively.	NA	Reported complication rate of TAA was still high and remained a significant clinical problem that could be severely hampering long-run clinical survival of TAA.
So et al,[29] 2022	Case series: comparison of rate of infection using SHS (group 1, N = 109) vs standard surgical attire (group 2, N = 151)	NA	260	NA	NA	NA	NA	There was no difference in revision rates between the 2 groups	The rate of PJI was 0.92% in group 1% and 2.6% in group 2.	The utility of SHS did not seem to influence the incidence of postoperative SSI or PJI.

(continued on next page)

Table 2
(continued)

Authors [Reference]	Type of Study	LoE	N	PROMs	Revision Rate	Reoperation Rate	Complication Rate	Conclusions
Yoon et al,[30] 2022	Case series: HINTEGRA TAA	IV	330 (364 ankles)	AOFAS, VAS, and AOS improved	43 ankles (28.5%) required revision procedures, with the most common reason being periprosthetic osteolysis (32 ankles [21.2%]).	NA	NA	HINTEGRA TAA gave satisfactory clinical outcomes, which were maintained at a FU of ≥10 y. The survival rate was 93.5%.
Baumfeld et al,[31] 2022	Case series: Corin-Zennith TAA	NA	29	AOFAS and VAS improved	NA	NA	24% cysts, 20.6% talar subsidence, 10.3% tibial subsidence	The Corin-Zennith TAA was a safe prosthesis for improving functional parameters.
Vesely et al,[32] 2022	Case series: Salto-Talaris TAA	IV	19	VAS improved	NA	10.5%,	21% according to the classification system reported by Glazebrook et al.	At a mean FU of 6.9 y (range, 3.5–12 y), there was 100% survivorship of the TAA
Vale et al,[33] 2023	SR	NA	4412	NA	NA	NA	The mean complication rate was 23.7% (2.4%–52%), mostly high-grade complications (35.6%).	Statistically significant positive correlation between high-grade and medium-grade complications and revision rates was found.

Author, year	Study type	Level	N			Results	Conclusions
Hermus et al,[34] 2022	Analysis of Arthroplasty Register	NA	810 patients (836 TAAs)	NA	NA	39 failures (4.7%): implant survival of 95.3% with a median FU of 38 mo.	Previous OCD treatment, BMI and age were associated with a higher risk for revision.
Rushing et al,[35] 2022	Case series: HO	III	90: 62 INFINITY, 28 CADENCE	NA	NA	HO incidence was 55.6% (56.5% for INFINITY, and 53.6% for CADENCE).	Similar incidence of HO after TAA with 2 different 4th generation TAAs was found.
Pfahl et al,[36] 2022	Case series: rTAA	NA	122	EFAS score improved	NA	The failure rate was 14.75%.	Adding procedures to correct alignment resulted in significantly lower revision rates
Othman et al,[37] 2022	Case series: soft tissue reconstruction of complicated TAA	IV	13	NA	NA	8 (61.5%) achieved prosthetic salvage, and 5 (38.5%) failed.	The prognosis for complicated TAA needing soft-tissue reconstruction remained poor, especially in individuals who presented with infected ankles.
Pfahl et al,[38] 2022	Case series: PJI after TAA treated with I&D and polyethylene exchange	NA	20	9%	40%	NA	I&D and polyethylene exchange had its limitations regarding infected TAA.

(continued on next page)

Table 2
(continued)

Authors [Reference]	Type of Study	LoE	N	PROMs	Revision Rate	Reoperation Rate	Complication Rate	Conclusions
Karzon et al,[39] 2022	IBM MarketScan database query	III	41,060	NA	NA	NA	NA	Yearly volumes and prevalence rates of primary TAA had augmented between 2009 and 2019.
Johnson et al,[40] 2022	Case series: effect of a TAL (N = 28) GR (N = 29) or no lengthening procedure (N = 55) during TAA on radiographic tibiopedal ROM.	III	112	NA	NA	NA	NA	Both TAL and GR augmented postoperative DF; however, this was accompanied by a reciprocal loss in PF. Minimal differences were found for ROM.
Stadler et al,[41] 2022	Case series: Salto Mobile Bearing TAA.	NA	171	AOFAS improved				Overall survival rate within the FU was 81.3% with any secondary surgery, 89.9% with revision, and 93.6% with reoperation as the endpoint.

Abbreviations: AA, ankle arthrodesis; AOFAS, American Orthopaedic Foot and Ankle Score; BMI, body mass index; DF, ankle dorsiflexion; EFAS, European Foot and Ankle Society; FAOS, Foot and Ankle Outcome Score; FU, follow-up; GR, gastrocnemius recession; HO, heterotopic ossification; I&D, irrigation and debridement; LoE, level of evidence; MA, meta-analysis; N, number of patients; NA, not available; OA, ankle osteoarthritis; OCD, osteochondritis dissecans; PF, plantar flexion; PJI, periprosthetic joint infection; ROM, range of motion; rTAA, revision total ankle arthroplasty; SHS, sterile helmet system; SF-12, Short form-12; SR, systematic review; SSI, surgical site infection; STAR, Scandinavian Total Ankle Replacement; TAL, tendo-Achilles lengthening; TAA, total ankle arthroplasty; VAS, Visual Analog Scale.

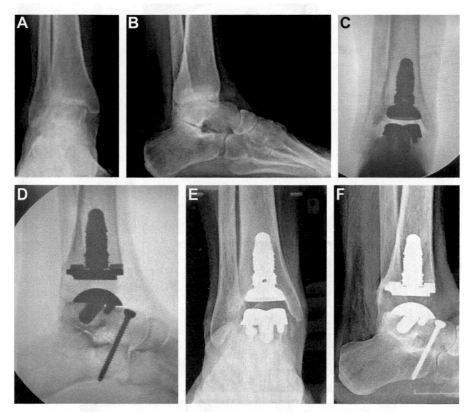

Fig. 3. (*A-F*) Woman with OA secondary to rheumatoid arthritis. She presented with disabling pain and joint stiffness with joint ROM less than 10°: (*A*) Preoperative AP radiograph showing severe degenerative changes in tibiotalar joint with correct alignment; (*B*) Preoperative lateral image showing severe joint impingement and tibiotalar and subtalar OA; (*C*) Intraoperative AP radiograph used to confirm the correct alignment and position of the tibial and talar components of an INBONE 2 (Wright) TAA; (*D*) Intraoperative lateral image showing correct tibial coverage with the prosthetic components and subtalar arthrodesis with a 4.5 mm lag screw; (*E*) AP radiograph 5 years after implantation of the TAA; (*F*) Lateral image of the TAA showing its good evolution 5 years after surgery. AP, anteroposterior; OA, osteoarthritis; ROM, range of motion; TAA, total ankle arthroplasty.

(<1% vs 2%), and below-knee amputation (<1% vs 5%) (*P* < .001 for all). Older age predicted lower revision risk after TAA, but age did not predict revision after AA. Although women were less likely to undergo revision after AA,[42] sex did not predict revision after TAA. The 2-year adjusted revision risk was 6% after TAA and 8% after AA. This difference was not statistically significant. Older age was a predictor of a lower revision risk after TAA.

In a systematic review, Gajebasia and colleagues compared the functional outcomes of AA and TAA.[43] They evaluated 898 AAs and 1638 TAASs. The mean follow-up was 3.3 years (range 0.5–13 years). Patients undergoing AA had a mean age of 55.7 years (range 20–82) and those undergoing TAA had a mean age of 62.5 years (range 21–89). There was significant heterogeneity in the outcomes used. No significant difference could be found between the reported change in PROMs after TAA and AA. Some 29.3% of the PROMs and their subscores showed that TAA had

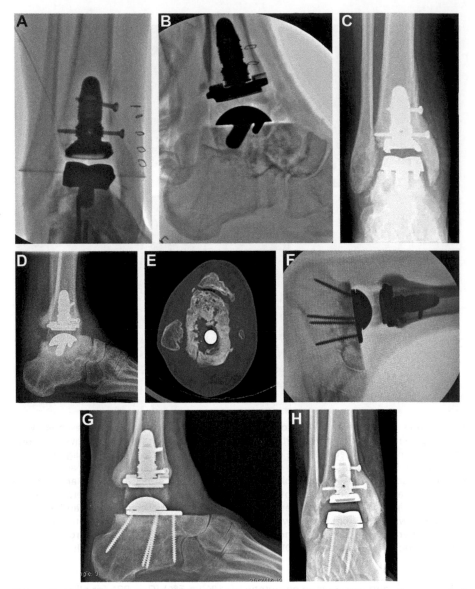

Fig. 4. (*A-H*) INBONE 2 (Wright Medical) TAA in a patient with ankle OA as a severe sequel of a talus fracture with partial necrosis: (*A*) Intraoperative AP radiograph showing correct alignment of the components. A tibial malleolus descent osteotomy and calcaneal valgus osteotomy were performed; (*B*) Intraoperative lateral image; (*C*) AP radiograph 1 year after prosthetic surgery. It shows that alignment was maintained and no mobilization of the tibial or talar components; (*D*) Two years after surgery, the patient began to have pain, swelling, and decreased joint ROM. Lateral radiograph showed loosening and subsidence of the talar component; (*E*) Axial CT image showing osteolysis around the stem of the talar component; (*F*) Intraoperative view of surgical revision and replacement of the talar component with an implant with an INVISION prosthetic talus platform and talocalcaneal screws (Wright Medical) compatible with INBONE 2 prosthetic tibial implant; (*G*) Lateral radiograph 5 years after prosthetic replacement surgery; (*H*) AP image 5 years after prosthetic replacement. AP, anteroposterior; CT, computed tomography; OA, osteoarthritis; ROM, range of motion; TAA, total ankle arthroplasty.

better results; 69% showed no significant difference; and only 2% showed that AA had better results. Most of the published studies found equality in PROMs after TAA and AA, albeit with relatively low study quality. Gajebasia and colleagues stated that randomized controlled studies were urgently needed to definitively demonstrate outcomes differences between AA and TAA.

Utilization Trends, In-hospital Length of Stay, Complications, and Costs

In a level III of evidence study, Tucker and colleagues evaluated utilization trends of TAA and AA and compared cost and complications. Medicare patients with a diagnosis of ankle OA were reviewed.[44] The investigators identified 673,789 patients with ankle OA. A total of 19,120 patients underwent an AA and 9059 had a TAA. While AA rates remained relatively constant, although slightly decreasing with 2080 performed in 2005 and 1823 performed in 2014, TAA rates nearly quadrupled. The mean cost associated with TAA was $12,559.12 compared with $6962.99 for AA ($P < .001$). Overall complication rates were 25% in the AA group with a revision rate of 16% compared with 15% and 11%, respectively, in the TAA group ($P < .001$). Individuals younger than 65 years had higher complication and revision rates. TAA became an increasingly popular option for the treatment of advanced ankle OA. In this study, TAA demonstrated lower revision and complication rates than AA. However, TAA was the far more expensive treatment option.[44]

Gordon and colleagues used the PearlDiver claims database from 2010 to 2019 to compare demographics and utilization of both surgical techniques (AA and TAA), in-hospital length of stay (LOS), and costs.[45] In total, 14,248 patients underwent primary TAA (n = 5544) or AA (n = 8704). The patients operated on with AA were, in general, younger (<60 years) and with a higher burden of comorbidity stemming from hypertension, diabetes mellitus, obesity, and tobacco use than the patients operated on with TAA ($P < .0001$). During the study period, TAA utilization remained constant (912 vs 909 interventions; $P = .807$), whereas AA utilization decreased by 42.5% (1737 vs 998 interventions; $P = .0001$). The mean in-hospital LOS of patients operated on with TAA decreased (2.5 days vs 2 days, $P = .0004$), whereas that of those operated on with AA increased (2.6 days vs 3.5 days, $P = .0003$). Expenditures for both interventions decreased significantly (more than 50%) during the study period (TAA: $4559–$2156; AA: $4729–$1721; $P < .013$). From 2010 to 2019, TAA utilization remained constant, whereas AA utilization decreased by 42%.[45]

In another level III of evidence study, Paracha and colleagues used a nationwide administrative claims database to compare the demographics between TAAs and AAs and determine whether patients undergoing TAA had higher utilization rates, in-hospital LOS, and costs than patients undergoing AA.[46] They queried the PearlDiver nationwide claims database from 2005 through December 2013 to identify patients who underwent TAA or primary AA for ankle and foot OA. Age, sex, geographic distribution, and Elixhauser Comorbidity Index (ECI) were compared between TAA and AA. The annual costs of both surgical techniques during the study period were also evaluated. A total of 21,433 patients undergoing primary TAA (n = 7126) and AA (n = 14,307) surgery were included. Those undergoing TAA had significantly higher ECI for arrythmias, congestive heart failure, diabetes mellitus, electrolyte/fluid disorders, and iron deficiency anemia than those undergoing AA ($P < .001$). From 2005 to 2013, the utilization of TAA increased from 21% to 49% ($P < .0001$). There was a greater reduction of in-hospital LOS for TAA than for AA (2.15 days vs 3.11 days, $P < .0001$). TAA reimbursements remained stable; however, the cost per individual increased significantly from $40,203.48 in 2005 to doubling by the end of 2013 to $86,208.59 ($P < .0001$). This study demonstrated greater use of TAA than AA, showing a decrease in in-hospital LOS and an increase in cost of care, with stagnant reimbursement rates.[46]

Brodeur and colleagues, also with level III evidence, studied trends in TAA and AA for ankle OA in New York State from 2009 to 2018 to determine whether patients' demographics had any bearing on the selection of surgical technique, the utilization of each, and their complication rates.[47] Individuals aged 40 years or older were identified using the International Classification of Diseases, Ninth and Tenth Revisions, Clinical Modification diagnosis and procedure codes for ankle OA, AA, and TAA in the New York State Cooperative Planning and Research System database from 2009 to 2018. A trend analysis was conducted over time. AA increased by 25%, while TAA increased by 757%. African American race, federal insurance, workers compensation, presence of comorbidities, and higher social deprivation were associated with higher odds of undergoing AA than TAA. Compared with TAA, AA was associated with higher rates of readmission, surgical site infection (SSI), acute renal failure, cellulitis, urinary tract infection, and deep vein thrombosis. The volume of TAA increased substantially without a decrease in the volume of AA, suggesting that TAA might have been used selectively for a different group of patients than AA. Despite the increase in TAA, certain groups of patients, such as those from minority populations, federal insurance, and from areas of high social deprivation, were more likely to undergo AA.[47]

Gait and Stair Ascent

With level III of evidence, Sanders and colleagues compared 3-dimensional foot and ankle kinetics and kinematics of the foot and ankle and determined the ankle power generated during level walking and stair climbing between patients with TAA and AA.[48] Ten patients operated on with TAA with a modern fixed-bearing ankle prosthesis and 10 patients operated on with AA were analyzed. The patients were matched for age, sex, body mass index, time since surgery, and preoperative diagnosis. The minimum follow-up was 2 years. The patients completed an instrumented 3-dimensional motion analysis while walking on level ground and during stair ascent. Sagittal range of motion (ROM) of the ankle was significantly greater in the TAA group (21.1 vs 14.7°, $P = .003$) during level walking. In addition, forefoot-tibia motion (25.3° vs 18.6°, $P = .015$) and hindfoot-tibia motion (15.4° vs 12.2°, $P = .022$) were significantly greater in the TAA group. During stair ascent, sagittal ankle ROM (25 vs 17.1°, $P = .026$), forefoot-tibia motion (27.6 vs 19.6°, $P = .017$), and hindfoot-tibia motion (16.8 vs 12°, $P = .012$) were greater. There were significant differences during level walking and stair ascent between patients with TAA and AA. Those with TAA generated greater peak plantar flexion power and sagittal motion within the foot and ankle than those with AA. Sanders and colleagues suggested further research was needed to evaluate biomechanical differences in the foot and ankle during other activities of daily living.[48]

The Impact of Coronal Plane Deformity in Ankle Osteoarthritis

In an observational level II of evidence trial, 224 patients treated for advanced ankle OA were studied. Of 112 patients followed for more than 2 years, 48 (19 AAs, 29 TAAs) had coronal plane deformity and were compared with 64 patients without coronal plane deformity (18 AAs, 46 TAAs), which was defined as greater than 10° of varus or valgus.[49] The ankle prostheses used had different internal constraints than intracomponent coronal plane tilting. The patients completed the Musculoskeletal Functional Assessment (MFA) and SF-36 before surgery and at 3, 6, 12, 12, 24, and 36 months after surgery. Outcome measures were the SF-36, MFA, reoperation rates, and pain scales. In patients with ankle deformity in the coronal plane, the median for the AA group was 19° and the median for the TAA group was 16.9°. In the coronal deformity group, there were 7 major reoperations: 2 in the AA group and 5 in the TAA group, all with the less constrained implant design. MFA, vitality, and SF-36 social function improved in all groups. At 2-year and 3-year follow-ups, patients without preoperative coronal deformity improved more than those without preoperative coronal deformity with both AA and TAA. There was no difference in improvement between patients with coronal deformity undergoing TAA or AA. That is, patients with and without coronal plane deformity can benefit from both TAA and AA, although those without preoperative deformity would be expected to improve more. At 3 years, no significant differences were found between AA and TAA in patient-reported outcomes among patients with advanced ankle OA and preoperative coronal plane deformity, regardless of whether they received an AA or TAA.[49]

Patients with Diabetes

In a systematic review and meta-analysis with level II evidence, Tarricone and colleagues compared the probability of major and minor complications between patients with and without diabetes operated on with TAAs and AAs.[50] The total number of surgical interventions was 26,287 (13,830 TAAs and 12,457 AAs). There was a significant relationship between patients with diabetes treated with AA and major complications, whereas no significant relationship was observed between patients with diabetes treated with TAA and major complications. This meta-analysis found that patients with diabetes have a significantly increased risk of major and minor complications when undergoing AA. However, no significant difference in major complications was observed between patients with and without diabetes who underwent TAA.[50]

Knee Kinetics and Kinematics

Roney and colleagues evaluated whether patients with TAA and AA had altered biomechanics related to the onset and progression of knee OA.[51] The knee adduction moment (KAM), a surrogate measure for the mechanical load experienced in the medial tibiofemoral compartment, was used because it is related to the onset and progression of knee OA. At least 2 years postoperatively, instrumented 3-dimensional walking gait was recorded in 10 patients with TAA and 10 patients with AA at self-selected walking speeds. The patients with TAA had either a Salto Talaris prosthesis or an INBONE prosthesis. Mean first and second peak KAM (Nm/kg), KAM impulse (Nm-s/kg), and ROM were calculated in the affected and unaffected limbs of each patient. There were no significant differences in the first and second peak KAM, knee impulse, or ROM in any plane between unaffected and affected limbs, or between TAA and AA. It appeared that in the short term, neither TAA nor AA significantly affected ipsilateral knee kinetics or KAMs. Roney and colleagues suggested that their study highlighted the importance of further investigating these parameters in larger groups of patients and with longer follow-up to determine whether treatment of advanced ankle OA affects the incidence or progression of ipsilateral KAM.[51]

Complications and Reoperations

Using a large database population (PearlDiver, www.pearldiverinc.com, Colorado Springs, CO, USA), Sambandam and colleagues analyzed the differences between AA and TAA in a matched sample of patients in terms of 30-day and 1-year complication and reoperation rates.[52] Using Current Procedural Terminology, patients operated on for TAA and AA were identified. After matching the TAA and AA groups based on confounding variables, such as diabetes, smoking, obesity, and comorbidities scores, differences in 30-day and 1-year complication rates and 1-year reoperation rates were assessed in both groups. There were 1287 patients in each group, with no significant differences in the male/female ratio. Within each group, 430 patients had diabetes, 102 were smokers, and 543 had obesity. The rate of SSI and wound dehiscence was higher at 30 days in the AA group. Some 63% of the complications occurred at 30 days. The AA group showed a higher rate of SSI, wound dehiscence, mechanical complications, and pneumonia at 1 year. The reoperation rate was also higher in the AA group at 1 year. Compared with TAA, AA was associated with a higher rate of local and systemic complications at 30 days and at 1 year, along with a higher reoperation rate at 1 year. Most complications occurred after 30 days, which is why Sambandam and colleagues stated that studies reporting 30-day complications of AA or TAA might underestimate true complication rates.[52]

Ross and colleagues found that patients with AA showed significantly higher percentages of at least 1 frequent joint complication at 90 days (19% vs 13%), 1 year (26% vs 15%), and 2 years (27% vs 16%) postoperatively. These results included higher percentages of adjacent fusion or osteotomy procedures, periprosthetic fractures, and hardware removal at each postoperative follow-up. Rates of infection were similar at 2 years postoperatively (4.3% vs 4.2%).[53]

PATIENTS' POINT OF VIEW ON THE LONG-TERM RESULTS

In a level IV of evidence study, Deleu and colleagues compared the results of TAA, TT arthrodesis, and TTC arthrodesis from the point of view of the operated patients. They proposed 2 hypotheses: that TAA would lead to better results than TT arthrodesis; and that TT arthrodesis would lead to better results than TTC arthrodesis.[54] They conducted a retrospective study including TAA, TT arthrodesis, and TTC arthrodesis performed in their hospital from 2010 to 2017. The results were compared using PROMs (Foot Function Index, FAOS, and SF-12). Fifty-one patients were included in the TAA group, 50 in the TT arthrodesis group, and 51 in the TTC arthrodesis group. The mean follow-up was 46 months. The TAA group performed better than the TT group in terms of Foot Function Index score and satisfaction, thus confirming the first hypothesis. On the other hand, no significant differences were found between the TT group and the TTC group, invalidating the second hypothesis. Deleu and colleagues stated that although it is difficult to compare surgeries with different indications, it was surprising to find that the patients' perceived recovery state, deviating from the usual clinical and radiological results, was relatively similar.[54]

SUMMARY

Several publications have found that the utilization rates of TAA have increased in recent years while those of AA have decreased. Regarding PROMs, in general, no differences were found between TAA and AA, although both interventions improved PROMs with respect to the preoperative situation. That is, both interventions (AA and TAA) are effective in terms of improving preoperative symptoms due to advanced ankle OA. On the other hand, 1 study observed that complication rates at 3 months, 1 year, and 2 years were higher after AA than after TAA (13%, 15%, and 16%, respectively). However, infection rates were similar (about 4%). In another study, the complication rate after AA was 25% versus 15% after TAA, and the revision rate was 16% after AA versus 11% after TAA. In short, it seems that TAA currently offers the same PROMs as AA, but with a lower percentage of complications, revisions, and reoperations in some published series. To definitively determine which operation is more Tsuitable in advanced ankle OA, more and better designed studies are required, given that the results published thus far do not allow us to determine which of the 2 interventions is more appropriate. The principal limitation of this article is that the selection of studies was subjective, that is, those that we deemed most directly related to the title of the article were chosen. Therefore, it is possible that some important articles were not included. This article is not a systematic review of the literature, but a narrative review of the articles we found most interesting. In addition, only the results of AA and TAA in the year 2022 were analyzed, and the comparative results between AA and TAA in the years 2021 and 2022.

CLINICS CARE POINTS

- When conservative treatment (analgesics, anti-inflammatory drugs, canes, unloading orthoses), alone or in combination with intraarticular injections of corticosterolds or hyaluronic acid and joint-preserving surgical treatment (arthroscopic debridement, realignment osteotomy, distraction arthroplasty), fails in patients with painful, advanced-stage ankle osteoarthritis (OA), there are 2 surgical options that do not preserve the joint: tibiotalar (TT) arthrodesis (ankle arthrodesis [AA]) or total ankle arthroplasty (TAA).

- Both interventions (AA and TAA) are effective in terms of improving preoperative symptoms due to advanced ankle OA.

- Regarding PROMs, no differences have been found between TAA and AA.

- TAA seems to offer a lower percentage of complications, revisions and reoperations.

- However, to definitively determine which operation is more suitable, more and better designed studies are required.

DISCLOSURE

The authors have nothing to disclose.

REFERENCES

1. Haddad SL, Coetzee JC, Estok R, et al. Intermediate and long-term outcomes of total ankle arthroplasty and ankle arthrodesis: a systematic review of the literature. J Bone Joint Surg Am 2007;89:1899–905.
2. Watts DT, Moosa A, Elahi Z, et al. Comparing the results of total ankle arthroplasty vs tibiotalar fusion (ankle arthrodesis) in patients with ankle osteoarthritis since 2006 to 2020: a systematic review. Arch Bone Jt Surg 2022;10:470–9.
3. Stołtny T, Dugieło B, Pasek J, et al. Tibiotalocalcaneal arthrodesis in osteoarthritis deformation of ankle and subtalar joint: evaluation of treatment results. J Foot Ankle Surg 2022;61:205–11.
4. Patel S, Baker L, Perez J, et al. Risk factors for nonunion following tibiotalocalcaneal arthrodesis: a systematic review and meta-analysis. Foot Ankle Surg 2022; 28:7–13.
5. van den Heuvel SBM, Penning D, Schepers T. Open ankle arthrodesis: a retrospective analysis comparing different fixation methods. J Foot Ankle Surg 2022;61: 233–8.
6. Martinelli N, Bianchi A, Raggi G, et al. Open versus arthroscopic ankle arthrodesis in high-risk patients: a comparative study. Int Orthop 2022;46:515–21.
7. Morasiewicz P, Dejnek M, Orzechowski W, et al. Subjective and objective outcomes of ankle joint arthrodesis with either Ilizarov or internal fixation. J Foot Ankle Surg 2023;62(1):39–44.

8. Shah AB, Davis W, Littlefield ZL, et al. Patient and surgical factors affecting fusion rates after arthroscopic and open ankle fusion: a review of a high-risk cohort. Indian J Orthop 2022;56:1217–26.

9. Li B, Wang S, Li Q, et al. Effectiveness of Ilizarov ankle arthrodesis in the treatment of end-stage varus ankle osteoarthritis: a retrospective study. Orthop Surg 2022;14:937–45.

10. Wong LH, Chrea B, Meeker JE, et al. Factors associated with nonunion and infection following ankle arthrodesis using a large claims database: who has elevated risk? Foot Ankle Orthop 2022;7. 24730114221101617.

11. Coye TL, Tirabassi N, Foote CM, et al. An umbrella systematic review and meta-analysis of systematic reviews on the topic of foot and ankle arthrodesis nonunion rates. J Foot Ankle Surg 2022. https://doi.org/10.1053/j.jfas.2022.04.012.

12. Chalak A, Singh S, Ghodke A, et al. Ilizarov ankle arthrodesis: a simple salvage solution for failed and neglected ankle fractures. Indian J Orthop 2022;56: 1587–93.

13. Fadhel WB, Taieb L, Villain B, et al. Outcomes after primary ankle arthrodesis in recent fractures of the distal end of the tibia in the elderly: a systematic review. Int Orthop 2022;46:1405–12.

14. Abuhantash M, Veljkovic A, Wing K, et al. Arthroscopic versus open ankle arthrodesis: a 5-year follow up. J Bone Joint Surg Am 2022;104:1197–203.

15. Reinke C, Lotzien S, Yilmaz E, et al. Tibiocalcaneal arthrodesis using the Ilizarov fixator in compromised hosts: an analysis of 19 patients. Arch Orthop Trauma Surg 2022;142:1359–66.

16. Cifaldi A, Thompson M, Abicht B. Tibiotalocalcaneal arthrodesis with structural allograft for management of large osseous defects of the hindfoot and ankle: a systematic review and meta-analysis. J Foot Ankle Surg 2022;61:900–6.

17. Liu T, Dong SJ, Li WL, et al. Ankle arthrodesis combined with mosaic bone autograft transplantation for end-stage ankle osteoarthritis with large cysts of talar dome. J Foot Ankle Surg 2022;61:932–7.

18. Mehdi N, Lintz F, Alsafi M, et al. Revision tibiotalar arthrodesis with posterior iliac autograft after failed arthroplasty: a matched comparative study with primary ankle arthrodeses. Orthop Traumatol Surg Res 2022;108:103269.

19. Loveday DT, Baskaran D, Salmasi MY, et al. The 15 year ankle arthroplasty experience in a university hospital. Foot Ankle Surg 2022;28:217–21.

20. Hauer G, Hofer R, Kessler M, et al. Revision rates after total ankle replacement: a comparison of clinical studies and arthroplasty registers. Foot Ankle Int 2022;43: 176–85.

21. Maccario C, Paoli T, Romano F, et al. Transfibular total ankle arthroplasty: a new reliable procedure at five-year follow-up. Bone Joint Lett J 2022;104-B:472–8.

22. Best MJ, Nguyen S, Shafiq B, et al. Risk factors for complications, longer hospital stay, and readmission after total ankle arthroplasty. Foot Ankle Spec 2022;15: 142–9.

23. Dagneaux L, Nogue E, Mathieu J, et al. Survivorship of 4,748 contemporary total ankle replacements from the French discharge records database. J Bone Joint Surg Am 2022;104:684–92.

24. Gagne OJ, Day J, Kim J, et al. Midterm survivorship of the INBONE II total ankle arthroplasty. Foot Ankle Int 2022;43:628–36.

25. Mo K, Ficke JR. The most-cited ankle arthroplasty implant articles. Foot Ankle Orthop 2022;7. 24730114221103862.

26. Consul DW, Chu A, Langan TM, et al. Total ankle arthroplasty survivorship, complication, and revision rates in patients younger than 55 years. Foot Ankle Spec 2022;15:283–90.

27. Shah JA, Schwartz AM, Farley KX, et al. Projections and epidemiology of total ankle and revision total ankle arthroplasty in the United States to 2030. Foot Ankle Spec 2022. https://doi.org/10.1177/19386400221109420. 19386400221109420.

28. Hermus JP, Voesenek JA, van Gansewinkel EHE, et al. Complications following total ankle arthroplasty: A systematic literature review and meta-analysis. Foot Ankle Surg 2022;28(8):1183–93.

29. So E, Juels CA, Seidenstricker C, et al. Postoperative infection rates after total ankle arthroplasty: a comparison with and without the use of a surgical helmet system. J Foot Ankle Surg 2022;61:802–6.

30. Yoon YK, Park KH, Park JH, et al. Long-term clinical outcomes and implant survivorship of 151 total ankle arthroplasties using the HINTEGRA prosthesis: a minimum 10-year follow-up. J Bone Joint Surg Am 2022;104:1483–91.

31. Baumfeld D, Baumfeld T, Rezende RF, et al. Corin ankle arthroplasty: case-series. Foot Ankle Surg 2022;28:745–9.

32. Vesely BD, King MA, Scott AT. Intermediate to long-term follow-up of the Salto Talaris fixed-bearing total ankle prosthesis. Foot Ankle Spec 2022. https://doi.org/10.1177/19386400221118495. 19386400221118495.

33. Vale C, Almeida JF, Pereira B, et al. Complications after total ankle arthroplasty- A systematic review. Foot Ankle Surg 2023;29(1):32–8.

34. Hermus JPS, van Kuijk SMJ, Spekenbrink-Spooren A, et al. Risk factors for total ankle arthroplasty failure: a Dutch Arthroplasty Register study. Foot Ankle Surg 2022;28:883–6.

35. Rushing CJ, Steriovski J, Hyer CF, et al. Heterotopic ossification following total ankle arthroplasty with fourth-generation prostheses. Foot Ankle Spec 2022;15:448–55.

36. Pfahl K, Röser A, Eder J, et al. Failure rates and patient-reported outcomes of revision of total ankle arthroplasty. Arch Orthop Trauma Surg 2022. https://doi.org/10.1007/s00402-022-04657-1.

37. Othman S, Colen DL, Azoury SC, et al. Soft-tissue reconstruction of complicated total ankle arthroplasty. Foot Ankle Spec 2022;15:464–71.

38. Pfahl K, Röser A, Gottschalk O, et al. Common bacteria and treatment options for the acute and chronic infection of the total ankle arthroplasty. Foot Ankle Surg 2022;28:1008–13.

39. Karzon AL, Kadakia RJ, Coleman MM, et al. The rise of total ankle arthroplasty use: a database analysis describing case volumes and incidence trends in the United States between 2009 and 2019. Foot Ankle Int 2022;43:1501–10.

40. Johnson LG, Fletcher AN, Wu CJ, et al. Tibiopedal motion following tondo-Achilles lengthening or gastrocnemius recession in total ankle replacement: a comparative cohort study. Foot Ankle Int 2022;43(12):1622–30.

41. Stadler C, Stöbich M, Ruhs B, et al. Intermediate to long-term clinical outcomes and survival analysis of the Salto Mobile Bearing total ankle prothesis. Arch Orthop Trauma Surg 2022;142:3697 704.

42. Randsborg PH, Jiang H, Mao J, et al. Two-year revision rates in total ankle replacement versus ankle arthrodesis: a population-based propensity-score-matched comparison from New York State and California. JB JS Open Access 2022;7(2). e21.00136.

43. Gajebasia S, Jennison T, Blackstone J, et al. Patient reported outcome measures in ankle replacement versus ankle arthrodesis - A systematic review. Foot 2022; 51:101874.
44. Tucker WA, Barnds BL, Morris BL, et al. Nationwide analysis of total ankle replacement and ankle arthrodesis in Medicare patients: trends, complications, and cost. Foot Ankle Spec 2022;15:201–8.
45. Gordon AM, Lam AW, Golub IJ, et al. Comparison of patient demographics, utilization trends, and costs of total ankle arthroplasty and ankle fusion in the United States from 2010 to 2019. Arch Orthop Trauma Surg 2022. https://doi.org/10. 1007/s00402-022-04481-7.
46. Paracha N, Idrizi A, Gordon AM, et al. Utilization trends of total ankle arthroplasty and ankle fusion for tibiotalar osteoarthritis: a nationwide analysis of the United States population. Foot Ankle Spec 2022. https://doi.org/10.1177/1938640022 1110133. 19386400221110133.
47. Brodeur PG, Walsh DF, Modest JM, et al. Trends and reported complications in ankle arthroplasty and ankle arthrodesis in the State of New York, 2009-2018. Foot Ankle Orthop 2022;7(3). 24730114221117150.
48. Sanders AE, Kraszewski AP, Ellis SJ, et al. Differences in gait and stair ascent after total ankle arthroplasty and ankle arthrodesis. Foot Ankle Int 2021;42:347–55.
49. Johnson MD, Shofer JB, Hansen ST Jr, et al. The impact of coronal plane deformity on ankle arthrodesis and arthroplasty. Foot Ankle Int 2021;42:1294–302.
50. Tarricone A, Gee A, Chen S, et al. A systematic review and meta-analysis of total ankle arthroplasty or ankle arthrodesis for treatment of osteoarthritis in patients with diabetes. Foot Ankle Orthop 2022;7(3). 24730114221112955.
51. Roney AR, Kraszewski AP, Demetracopoulos CA, et al. Knee kinetics and kinematics in patients with ankle arthroplasty and ankle arthrodesis. HSS J 2022; 18:408–17.
52. Sambandam S, Serbin P, Riepen D, et al. Differences between total ankle replacement and ankle arthrodesis in post-operative complications and reoperations at 30 days and one year. Cureus 2022;14(9):e28703.
53. Ross BJ, Savage-Elliott I, Wu VJ, et al. Complications following total ankle arthroplasty versus ankle arthrodesis for primary ankle osteoarthritis. Foot Ankle Spec 2021. https://doi.org/10.1177/1938640020987741. 1938640020987741.
54. Deleu PA, Piron M, Leemrijse G, et al. Patients' point of view on the long-term results of total ankle arthroplasty, tibiotalar and tibiotalocalcaneal arthrodeses. Orthop Traumatol Surg Res 2022;108(7):103369.

Total Ankle Arthroplasty in Young Patients

M. Pierce Ebaugh, DO[a],*, William C. McGarvey, MD[b]

KEYWORDS

- Total ankle replacement • Ankle arthroplasty • Ankle arthrodesis
- Revision total ankle

KEY POINTS

- With continuing advancements in total ankle arthroplasty (TAA), it is quickly becoming the procedure of choice for older patients with end-stage ankle arthritis.
- Considerations of TAA versus ankle arthrodesis, TAA implant longevity, outcomes of revision TAA, and whether patients should be offered an arthrodesis with plans for conversion to arthroplasty may help elucidate whether pursuing ankle arthroplasty in a younger, more active population is the correct approach for surgeons.
- The traditional gold standard operative treatment for ankle arthritis has been arthrodesis.

INTRODUCTION

With continuing advancements in total ankle arthroplasty (TAA), it is quickly becoming the procedure of choice for older patients with end-stage ankle arthritis.[1–5] Unfortunately, due to its post-traumatic nature, ankle arthritis often plagues a younger population.[4,6] Multiple studies have been conducted on younger patients who have undergone TAA with promising results, but is it the procedure of choice?[2,7–10] Considerations of TAA versus ankle arthrodesis, TAA implant longevity, outcomes of revision TAA, and whether patients should be offered an arthrodesis with plans for conversion to arthroplasty may help elucidate whether pursuing ankle arthroplasty in a younger, more active population is the correct approach for surgeons.

FUSION VERSUS REPLACEMENT

The traditional gold standard operative treatment for ankle arthritis has been arthrodesis. Currents trends in older populations challenge this standard with dramatic

[a] Jewett Orthopedic Institute at Orlando Health, 1285 N Orange Avenue, Winter Park, FL 32789, USA; [b] Orthopedic Foot and Ankle Reconstruction, McGovern College of Medicine - University of Texas Health Science Center at Houston, 6400 Fannin, Suite 1700, Houston, TX 77030, USA
* Corresponding author.
E-mail address: mpebaugh@gmail.com

Foot Ankle Clin N Am 29 (2024) 53–67
https://doi.org/10.1016/j.fcl.2023.08.011
1083-7515/24/© 2023 Elsevier Inc. All rights reserved.
foot.theclinics.com

increases in replacement.[3] The effect of adjacent joint arthritis, gait changes, and reoperation/complication rates should be carefully examined and explained with shared decision making before pursuit of definitive treatment.

Hindfoot Arthritis Progression

Prevention of adjacent joint arthritis progression has often been a highlighted advantage of TAA. In a classic study, Coester and colleagues[11] followed 23 patients for a mean of 22 years following ankle arthrodesis radiographically analyzing ipsilateral and contralateral knee, ankle, and foot joints for arthritic progression. They found nearly all patients had significant radiographic evidence of arthritis in ipsilateral hindfoot joints when compared with the contralateral side. Additionally, the authors found their patients significantly limited by the ipsilateral foot pain they experienced. Interestingly, no significant knee or midfoot arthritis was appreciated by authors on the ipsilateral side.

Ling and colleagues[12] systematically reviewed a collective of 24 studies, noting clear biomechanical alteration of the natural ankle motion without direct correlation to hindfoot arthritic progression. However, the authors did relate clear evidence of adjacent joint arthritis with nearly some studies having nearly 100% prevalence of subtalar arthritis and 77% of talonavicular/calcaneocuboid joint arthritis.

Dekker and colleagues[13] analyzed 140 TAA patients at a mean follow-up of 6.5 years, evaluating patients on whether they had radiographic increase in their modified Kellgren Lawrence knee osteoarthritis grading. They discovered 73% of subtalar and 69% of talonavicular joints displayed no grade increase. A total of 11% of patients required a subsequent subtalar arthrodesis and 2% required a talonavicular arthrodesis, all of these patients had both clinically and radiographically significant progression of arthritis.

Gait Analysis

Maintenance of natural ankle functional motion is one of the main goals of TAA. For a younger and presumably more active patient, preservation of quality during their most active years is very important when considering the greater impact of end-stage ankle arthritis on physical, mental, and general health in comparison to more prevalent arthritis of other joints.[14]

Although many patients are often satisfied with their ankle arthrodesis, it has been objectively shown that these patients experience a more abnormal gait and hindfoot function when compared with TAA. Thomas and colleagues[15] compared 26 ankle arthrodesis patients at a mean of 44 months with a control group for gait abnormalities, American Foot and Ankle Society (AOFAS) hindfoot scoring, Ankle Osteoarthritis Scale (AOS), and a Musculoskeletal Outcomes Data Evaluation and Management System (MODEMS) questionnaire. They discovered significant differences in cadence and stride length between the groups along with significant decreases in hindfoot and midfoot motion. In addition, the authors noted a 15% prevalence of moderate to severe subtalar joint arthritis at the time of analysis.

In a landmark study, Flavin and colleagues[16] analyzed the gait of 14 TAA and 14 ankle arthrodesis patients with a control group. Using temporospatial evaluation, TAA patients displayed a greater walking velocity via increased cadence and stride length when compared with arthrodesis patients. Additionally, TAA patients maintained a more symmetric vertical ground reaction force which was closer to controls.

Perceived function after TAA has been shown to be related to maintained motion. In a study of 41 TAA patients and 27 arthrodesis patients, TAA patients displayed greater sagittal plane and talonavicular motion in addition to better pain relief and perceived postoperative function.[17] It should be noted, however, that this improved range of motion still contains contribution from the mid/hindfoot joints. Dekker and colleagues[13] analyzed 179 total ankle replacements and their range via flexion/extension radiographs. They found that the ankle accounted for 68% of the total arc of motion, which is approximately 12% less than clinically observed.

Reoperation Rates and Complications

When counseling young patients on decision-making between TAA and ankle arthrodesis, reoperation rates and complications should always be included as part of the discussion. Due to the young age of implantation, it is certainly more likely than not that the patient will experience future procedures on their ankle.

SooHoo and colleagues[18] analyzed 4705 ankle fusions and 480 TAA over a 10-year period (1995–2004) from the California hospital discharge database. At 5 years they found a 9% reoperation rate for TAA compared with only 5% for arthrodesis. Complications were even more prevalent, with 23% of TAA patients having experienced a complication compared with 11% with fusion. Rates of subtalar arthrodesis were significantly higher in the fusion group, however. In a study with current generation implants, Ross and colleagues[19] discovered reoperation rates for TAA at 1 and 2 years to be 17% and 20% respectively, while ankle arthrodesis patients through the same time interval had significantly higher rates of reoperation, 35% and 42%, respectively. Furthering their investigation, they reported ankle arthrodesis patients to exhibit significantly greater complications at years with 26.9% of patients experiencing a major complication versus 16.2% of TAA patients. Additionally, they found similar rates of deep infection at approximately 4% for both categories.[20]

A randomized controlled trial of 281 patients undergoing ankle arthrodesis versus TAA found greater risk of wound healing complication and nerve injuries in ankle replacement, with significantly higher rates of nonunion (7%) and thromboembolism at 52 weeks from surgery in arthrodesis patients. Post hoc analysis suggested superiority of TAA over fusion.[21]

SooHoo and colleagues[22] performed an expansion on their previous study including nearly twice as many TAA and ankle fusion patients (1280 and 8491, respectively), this time including patients from 2005 to 2010. With the inclusion of more modern techniques and protheses, TAA displayed lower rates of deep infection and hospital readmission, in addition to increased utilization.

Analysis of the presented data shows the significant improvement in TAA technique, implant design, and patient selection. Additionally, much of this data still contain antiquated implant designs compared with what is available to today's surgeons.

Patient Satisfaction

Perceived functional improvement and quality of life is arguably the most important metric when considering whether to fuse or replace a patient's ankle. In our discussion regarding these 2 procedures, there is ample evidence for superiority of TAA in prevention of hindfoot arthritis, gait, and complications; however, are these measures significantly perceptible to the patient?

Younger and colleagues[23] compiled patient pre- and postoperative expectations and satisfaction in those undergoing TAA and ankle arthrodesis. A total of 654 patients were analyzed at a mean of 61 months following surgery using MODEM scoring for patient satisfaction and AOS scale for function. The group concluded that patients undergoing TAA had higher preoperative expectations but these were more likely to be met than patients undergoing arthrodesis, and that TAA were more satisfied overall. Surgeons should also note that patients' expectations preoperatively correlated little with their AOS function, but their satisfaction correlated greatly with their postoperative function. Counseling should be provided to any patient whose expectations exceed the capability of the procedure.

Recently, a unique study evaluated 10 patients, each with a TAA and a contralateral ankle arthrodesis. Overall each reconstruction demonstrated advantages and disadvantages according to the patients; however, most patients articulated a preference for their TAA side.[24]

Sangeorzan and colleagues[25] compared patient-reported outcome measures (PROMs) at 4 years following TAA and arthrodesis. TAA displayed greater improvement in Foot and Ankle Ability Measure (FAAM) acitivities of daily living (ADLs) and sports in addition to 36-Item Short Form Health Survey (SF-36) scores. Interestingly, TAA patients had slightly worse pain in years 1 to 3 of their ankle when compared with fusion; however, this attenuated at 4 years. Expectedly, all improvements made at 2 years were maintained at 4 years.

Knowledge of the advantages and disadvantages of both procedures indicated for end-stage ankle arthritis is essential for the orthopedic surgeon when considering a possible ankle replacement in a younger patient. Shared decision-making at this crossroads helps patients define their expectation for each procedure. The longevity of ankle replacement must always be an essential part of this discussion; however, with new implant designs entering the market every year, this can be difficult to define for the patient.

TOTAL ANKLE ARTHROPLASTY IMPLANT DESIGN AND LONGEVITY

Upon consideration of TAA for a younger patient, part of the shared decision-making process involves implant longevity and eventual need for revision surgery. This is often a difficult question to answer, as currently we do not have long-term outcomes on the majority of minimal resection implants available today. However, extrapolation of older data can aid in the discussion.

A meta-analysis performed in 2007 on intermediate and long-term outcome and survivorship comparisons of total ankle replacement (TAR) versus arthrodesis, TAA had an overall 2% lower revision rate, a higher mean AOFAS hindfoot score, lower below knee amputation rates, along with similar percentages of excellent/good outcomes. Ten-year survival rates in this study were relatively poor at 77%. It is also important to note that this meta-analysis was performed on data published from 1998 to 2005, which includes many second-generation total ankle implant designs that are no longer in routine use today or have undergone significant design updates.[26]

Another meta-analysis by Zaidi and colleagues[27] evaluated 7942 TAAs from national joint registries and included 8 different total ankle designs. Following overall pooled analysis, they found a 10-year overall survival rate of 89% but found a lower failure rate of just 1.1% per year in those TAAs performed by a design surgeon. Once again, it is important to note that this study included protheses that are not currently a popular choice among surgeons, additionally it showed that surgeons who were more familiar with the implants (ie, design surgeons) produced a lower yearly failure rate.

Palanca and colleagues[28] retrospectively analyzed 84 STAR TAAs performed between 1998 and 2000, finding a 73% survival rate at 15 years; they also concluded that most patients whose ankle survived to 9 years were likely to have survivorship to 15 years. Although this is a single surgeon/institution study, it provides some of the longest term outcome data available for a currently used prothesis.

Analyzing European National Joint Registry data with application of Kaplan-Meier survivability curves and controlling for protheses that have either been removed from the market or fallen out of use, Roukis and Bartel[29] showed a 0.90 to 0.93 survival at 5 years in 5152 primary and 591 revision TAR. This provides an excellent overview of survivorship in more modern componentry, displaying improvement in technique and design across all surgeons, not just those involved in implant design.

It should be noted that in prior outdated implants, authors have found no significant difference in survivorship between popular implants at that time.[30] Additionally, a study of 533 TAAs with at least 5 years of follow-up demonstrated no increased revision or failure rates in younger patients.[31] Although we do not have long-term data on many of our current implants, we have been able to improve implant design and outcomes in the short term due to advancing technology. Patient specific instrumentation (PSI) is currently used in many of the modern TAA designs. The basis for this comes from knowledge of mechanical alignment advantages from our hip and knee arthroplasty colleagues. Goldberg and colleagues[32] have demonstrated in several studies the overwhelming need to approach ankle arthroplasty in terms of overall limb mechanical axis alignment. Assuming that the overall limb mechanical axis is equivalent to the tibia mechanical and anatomic axis is often incorrect in TAA patients due to the post-traumatic nature of the disease.[4] In patients with former trauma proximal to the tibiotalar joint, or significant knee osteoarthritis, the authors recommend that the surgeons relies on hip knee ankle alignment films to evaluate the entire mechanical axis of the limb.[32,33] This has strengthened the basis for PSI that is now found in many widely used TAAs, allowing for the surgeon to properly align the implant with the mechanical axis. Additionally, this group has provided insight into the value that PSI provides for proper rotation of the implant to avoid impingement. Prior implants using standard instrumentation were set off the medial gutter line rather than the transmalleolar axis. The authors displayed the great variability in ankle rotation in those with arthritis, and recommended using computed tomography scan/PSI to help set rotation in TAA.[34]

Most currently available TAA systems now offer ultrahigh-molecular-weight polyethylene with improved wear properties.[35] This helps TAA more closely match current use total hip (THA) and knee arthroplasty (TKA) systems in terms of polyethylene quality. In addition to attempting to match implant quality with our hip and knee colleagues, TAA implant design has advanced into revision arthroplasty systems when indicated (Stryker INVISION and Integra XT). This advancement was mirrored in total knee arthroplasty approximately 20 years ago, and caused a significant paradigm shift regarding patient age when considering total knee replacement.

TOTAL ANKLE ARTHROPLASTY REVISION OUTCOMES

With these considerations and the advent of revision protheses, there is a paradigm shift for many orthopedic foot and ankle surgeons that mirrors observations seen 2 decades prior in total knee arthroplasty. On improvement in revision prothesis componentry, orthopedic surgeons gained confidence in providing younger patients with tricompartmental knee arthrosis and arthroplasty knowing there were revision options for these patients as they aged.[36,37] Losina and colleagues[36] demonstrated an increase of 134% from 1999 to 2008 in the number of TKAs performed in the United States, with the greatest increase found in the 45 to 64 year age group. Authors pointed to the fact that the spike in the number of arthroplasties was not related to increasing obesity or population, suggesting an improvement in implant survivability confidence. A prior meta-analysis demonstrated revision total knee arthroplasty to be a safe and effective procedure with re-revision rates of only 12.9%. The advancement of revision TKA systems in the early 2000s allowed for relaxed indications for primary implantation into younger patients and those with more complex deformities.[37] The availability of revision componentry for TAA allows surgeons to consider ankle replacement for patients who will most likely require a revision secondary to chronologic or physiologic age.

Revision arthroplasty is not for the faint of heart, however (**Fig. 1**). Ellington and colleagues[38] reported on some of the earliest TAA revision surgery, retrospectively reviewing 41 patients who underwent revision of the Agility prothesis at a mean of 51 months following primary surgery. Follow-up time was an average of 49 months from revision with prosthesis retention of 83%, 5 patients being converted to fusion and 2 undergoing amputation. Hintermann and colleagues[39] followed 117 patients who underwent revision TAA at a mean of 4 years from primary surgery displaying a

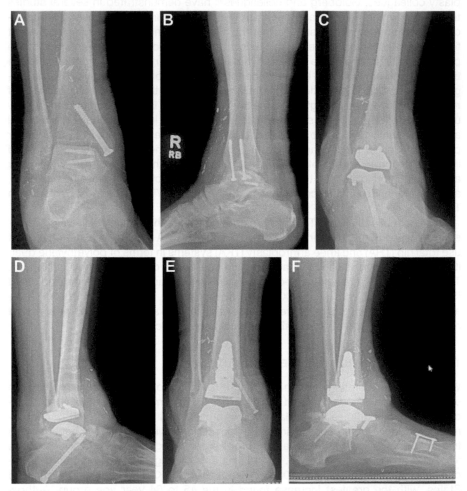

Fig. 1. A 42 year old man sustained a talus fracture during a work injury that resulted in post-traumatic ankle arthritis secondary to talus avascular necrosis and infection (*A, B*). He underwent total ankle arthroplasty with concurrent subtalar arthrodesis at an outside center that ultimately resulted in failure of tibial and talus components (*C, D*). He was then treated with revision total ankle arthroplasty with cement and metallic wedge augmentation of the remaining talus (*E, F*). (*Courtesy of* William C McGarvey MD.)

prothesis retention rate of 83% at 9 years from revision. After reviewing AOFAS scores, the authors concluded that intermediate follow-up results were comparable to primary surgery. Revisions are not without complications, with several studies showing rates of further surgery to be 17% and 26%.[39,40] Currently, there are no studies displaying long term outcomes with the novel revision systems previously mentioned. However, the Charlotte group has analyzed their mid-term outcomes of revision TAA using an intramedullary TAA implant. Eighteen TAAs at a mean of approximately 4 years from revision were evaluated, with nearly 22% of patients needing an operation at an average of 57 months postoperatively. Subsidence was prevalent with 38% of tibia and 55% of talus implants displaying change. Overall patients reported average outcomes, demonstrating a mean AOFAS score of 74 and foot function index (FFI) of 10.[41] In 29 TAAs at a mean of 3.2 years following revision arthroplasty, Lachman and colleagues[42] reinforced this finding with PROMs shown to be better following primary rather than revision surgery.

ANKLE ARTHRODESIS TAKEDOWN TO ARTHROPLASTY

In younger patients, many surgeons still defer to performing ankle arthrodesis for end-stage ankle arthritis. During the decision-making process, the possibility of future conversion of the arthrodesis to arthroplasty is often discussed. Although this is not a common procedure, it certainly has value in a patient with a painful or malaligned arthrodesis or in a patient with developing symptomatic arthritis (**Fig. 2**).[43–45]

Easley and colleagues[45] retrospectively analyzed 23 takedown TAAs at a mean follow-up of just under 3 years, with 12 of the ankles being performed for adjacent hindfoot osteoarthritis and the other 11 performed for subtalar or tibiotalar arthrodesis nonunion. There were significant improvements in visual analog scale (VAS) pain, SF-36, and Short Musculoskeletal Function Assessment; however, 13% of TAAs required revision due to subsidence. Additionally the authors found 70% of talus and 20% of tibia componentry to exhibit a degree of settling.[45]

A study of 77 patients with intermediate follow-up mean of 8.3 years exhibited an arguably better prothesis retention rate of 88%. The mean time to takedown from primary arthrodesis was 8.6 years, and the authors noted no significant difference in outcomes in terms of short-term versus long-term fusions. Patients continued to show range of motion improvement, gaining a mean of 20° at 25 months.[43]

Recently, Coetzee and colleagues[44] analyzed single surgeon outcomes of 51 takedown arthroplasties with a mean follow-up of 4.2 years. At final follow-up, patients had achieved a range of motion improvement of an average of 15.5° of dorsiflexion and 14.1° of plantarflexion. Patients enjoyed improvements in Veterans Rand Health Survey 12, AOS, and VAS pain scale. Only one patient underwent TAA removal following surgery at 12.7 months following TAA due to deep infection.[44]

The previous discussion is encouraging when considering the timeline for staging very young patients with ankle arthritis. Takedown arthroplasty is a viable consideration at a point even a decade following initial fusion, and for end-stage ankle arthritis patients who maybe in the 20s and 30s, a promising option to preserve ankle and hindfoot function into their 50s.

OUTCOMES OF YOUNGER PATIENTS UNDERGOING TOTAL ANKLE ARTHROPLASTY
Prior Studies

The main discussion point of our article centers around how younger patients perform in terms of longevity and outcomes with TAA. With often more active lifestyles and therefore greater expectations, performing an ankle replacement in younger patients

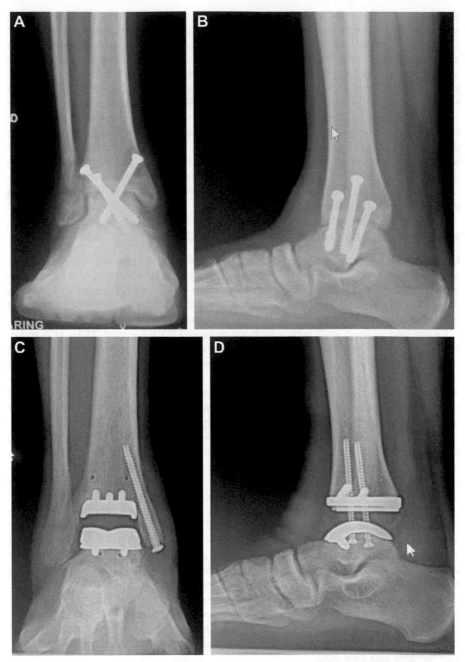

Fig. 2. Following an ankle fracture that progressed to post-traumatic arthritis, a 37 year old man underwent an ankle arthrodesis that resulted in nonunion (*A, B*). He then elected for takedown total ankle arthroplasty rather than revision arthrodesis (*C, D*). (Courtesy Willaim C McGarvey MD.)

is demanding and requires a thorough understanding of the limitations of the procedures to produce patient expectations in line with probable outcomes (**Fig. 3**).

The earliest study analyzing outcomes of TAA in younger patients was performed by Kofoed and Lundberg-Jensen,[46] who prospectively followed 100 TAAs (30 less than 50 years, 70 >50 years) annually for 15 years. The STAR total ankle prosthesis (previously STRYKER, now DJO GLOBAL) was used exclusively, with implantation occurring from years 1981 to 1996. In the less than 50 year old patient group, survivability was 86.7% with 1 patient being revised and 3 others being converted to arthrodesis. The older than 50 years patient group performed slightly, but not significantly better with a survivability of 88.5% with 4 patients being revised and another 4 being converted to arthrodesis. The mean time to failure was comparable at 5 years in less than 50 years group and 5.5 in the greater than 50 years group. Pain and functional scoring did not differ significantly between the 2 groups; however, the younger group displayed worse mobility scoring. The authors contributed this to 6 specific cases where the patients had complete hindfoot fusions distal to the ankle or dorsiflexion paresis.

Using now antiquated, third-generation componentry, Rodrigues-Pinto and colleagues[47] analyzed 31 patients aged less than 50 years with 72 patients aged greater than 50 years who underwent primary TAA with average follow-ups of 39 months and 42, respectively. No differences were found in survivorship rates (both 93%) or range

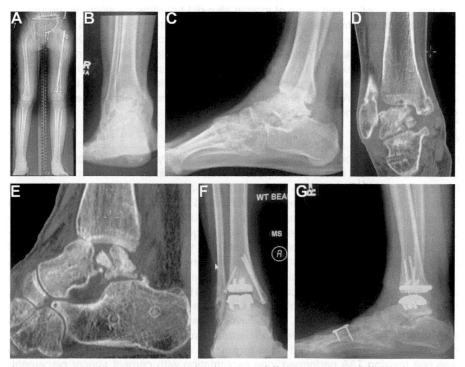

Fig. 3. A 24 year old woman sustained polytrauma following a 5 story fall off of a rooftop. Her injuries also resulted in right varus post-traumatic ankle and subtalar joint arthritis (A–C). Her arthritic ankle was complicated by a nonunited posterior body of the talus fracture (D, E). After extensive consultation and explanations of potential risks and benefits, she elected to proceed with total ankle arthroplasty with associated procedures (F, G). (*Courtesy of* William C McGarvey MD.)

of motion (both significantly improved) between the groups. The younger group trended toward less minor complications, with no significant differences in major complications. Interestingly, both groups also displayed significant improvement in AOFAS score, the less than 50 year age group demonstrated significantly greater improvement, scoring 93.5 versus 89.8.

In the only study employing gait analysis, Tenenbaum and colleagues[2] retrospectively evaluated 21 patients aged greater than 70 years with 21 patients aged 50 to 60 years who underwent TAA and compared both clinical (visual analog scale for pain, SF-36, AOFAS score) and 3-dimensional gait analysis at 2 weeks prior to TAA and then again at a minimum of 2 years postoperatively. There were no significant differences in clinical or gait analysis values between the 2 groups, both of which enjoyed significant improvements over preoperative numbers. Interestingly, the younger group showed greater improvements in overall ankle, knee, and hip range of motion. Although not mentioned by the authors, this could be related to more genetic and age-related osteoarthritis found in the hip and knee.

In a significantly larger prospective study, Demetracopoulos and colleagues[9] identified 3 groups of TAA patients, less than 55 years, 55 to 70 years, and greater than 70 years with 81, 221, 93 patients in each group, respectively. The average follow-up was 3.5 years. They found the less than 55 year age group displayed the greatest improvement in AOFAS and SF-36 scores without differences in wound complications, revisions, and need for reoperation between the groups. It should be noted that physical function and range of motion also did not differ between the groups.

Another retrospective analysis of outcomes on 51 patients aged less than 55 year old who underwent primary TAA with a mean follow-up of 31 months. Overall implant survivorship was 94%, with 7 patients needing a return trip to the operating room. Only 3 patients required explantation with revision arthroplasty or conversion to arthrodesis.[8] These outcomes were mirrored by Usuelli and colleagues,[10] who found greater improvement in AOFAS score and survivorship at 2 years in their younger cohort (age ≤50 years) using a mobile-bearing prosthesis.

Our Cohort

In the youngest cohort to date, we retrospectively analyzed 41 patients (21 females and 20 males) with at least 1 year of post clinical follow-up as well as recording patient PROMs via telephone interview on 31 of these patients. Included measures utilized consisted of SF-36, Patient- Reported Outcomes Measurement Information System Global Health, and Sickness Impact Profile Ambulation. The functional outcomes in our study sample were compared with age- and gender-matched norms from a general US population, and 95% confidence intervals were calculated for each functional outcome mean. Student's t test was used for continuous variables, and χ^2 analysis was used for categorical variables. Our mean age at surgery was 39.7 year old with average radiographic and clinical follow-ups of 31.2 and 51.6 months, respectively, following primary total ankle replacement. Our mean follow-up for outcomes respondents was 59.7 months. Overall, our survivorship was comparable to previous studies at 93%. Preoperatively, 26 ankles had neutral coronal plane alignment (5 or less degrees of varus or valgus), 9 had varus alignment, and 6 had valgus alignment. There was one revision TAA performed, one explantation with cement spacer placement, and one below-knee amputation. The majority of patients were obese with an average body mass index (BMI) of 31.2, patient selection included a large number of tobacco users (26.8%), and several patients diagnosed with diabetes mellitus (9.8%). To our knowledge, we are the first to display reported outcomes scores in patients with a mean age less than 40 years who underwent a TAA. Despite their young age and often increased demands, patient responders displayed improved well-being, with 81% reporting a good/very good/excellent quality of life, 81% reporting return to full employment and performing their duties without difficulty, and 84% stating they resumed all normal social activities. Few were hindered by fatigue (5/31), and the majority could ambulate frequently for long periods of time (61%). Most patients (87%) stated that they would have a TAA again, and of the 4 respondents who would have chosen other means of care, 3 still maintained the ability to ambulate frequently for long distances and stated they enjoyed a good or very good quality of life. The strengths of our data set include the youngest mean age found among prior studies (39.7 years with all patients aged <50 years) along with the longest reported average clinical follow-up of 51.6 months for all 41 patients and nearly 5 years (59.7 months) for outcomes respondents.[7] Our study contains notable limitations. Because of the patient population being extrapolated from a tertiary care referral trauma center, the population is transient to a degree, creating follow-up inconsistencies. Additionally, our patients have heterogeneity in the etiology of ankle arthritis (eg, ankle fractures, talus fractures, tibial plafond fractures, arthrodesis takedown, rheumatoid arthritis, and hemophilia). We reported on a modest number of patients making it difficult to weigh complete practice management changes from the data set. Finally using telephone interviews is not as effective in controlling bias in comparison to computer reported versions. The "yes" or "no" nature of the questions fails to enlighten certain patient responses, such as why the 3 patients who reported they would not have a TAA again stated they still had a good quality of life and could ambulate to long distances.

Discussion

The focus of this article and the insight of our study shows outcomes related to ambulation, satisfaction, pain, employment, social, and emotional well-being as perceived by a younger patient with a TAA. This is strengthened by the lack of difference found between age/gender-matched norms in the general population when compared with our cohort. Knowing that a younger patient has increased demands in these outcome areas, surgeons have more information to relay to patients when having a shared decision-making discussion in the clinic with a young patient plagued by end stage ankle arthritis. Our study and the previously included articles bolster the ability of surgeons to provide progressive care to patients; however, as with many difficult situations in the orthopedic field, it requires many more studies with larger patient numbers to conclude a paradigm or standard change should be made.

Although a prior study of 538 TAAs failed to find age as correlating demographic to early failure, many orthopedic surgeons are hesitant with consideration of placing a TAA into a younger, demanding patient.[31] This remains a valid thought process as our hip and knee colleagues have identified age to be a greater determinate on prothesis survival. Bayliss and colleagues[48] used a large online registry to identify 63,158 THA and 54,276 TKA patients followed for a maximum of 20 years, finding a 5% risk of revision for those aged greater than 70 years, yet a dramatic increase to 35% risk of revision for men in their 50s. This is coupled with the fact that TAA patient-reported outcomes still lag slightly behind hip and knee patients.

Five-year PROMs of THA, TKA, and TAA in patients with mean ages greater than 60 years showed that TAA displayed similar improvements when compared with hip and knee in terms of pain relief, satisfaction with the procedure, return to activities of daily living, and mental health. However, they performed worse in terms of stiffness, function, and return to recreational activities.[49] Our findings mirror this, with 58% of patients stating that they were limited in vigorous activities.

SUMMARY

As surgeons, we are beginning to recognize the desire for some younger patients to undergo total ankle replacement due to potential functional and preventive measures found with the procedure. In the current age of mass information and marketing via the internet and social media, their self-education must be tempered by a shared decision-making process with their provider that includes peer reviewed literature and procedural expectations/limitations. Keeping in mind all of this, we maintain that TAA is a viable option for a young patient in the correctly optimized setting in the effort to eliminate and/or reduce their pain while providing improved gait and delaying the onset of hindfoot arthritis.[4,16,18] As componentry evolves, we hope surgeons continue to expand the bank of literature of total ankle replacement in the younger patient.

CLINICS CARE POINTS

- A thorough pre operative evaluation of each patient that is being considered for total ankle arthroplasty should be undertaken.
- Mindfulness of risk factors including vascular status, tobacco use, diabetes mellitus, prior trauma should be closely analyzed prior to arthroplasty.

DISCLOSURE

W.C. McGarvey is a paid consultant and royalty bearing surgeon for Stryker/Wright medical.

REFERENCES

1. Berlet GC, Brandão RA, Consul D, et al. Short- to Midterm Follow-up of Cemented Total Ankle Replacement Using the INBONE II: A Retrospective Chart Review. Foot Ankle Spec 2021;14(4):302–11.
2. Tenenbaum S, Bariteau J, Coleman S, et al. Functional and clinical outcomes of total ankle arthroplasty in elderly compared to younger patients. Foot Ankle Surg 2017;23(2):102–7.
3. Raikin SM, Rasouli MR, Espandar R, et al. Trends in treatment of advanced ankle arthropathy by total ankle replacement or ankle fusion. Foot Ankle Int 2014;35(3):216–24.
4. Saltzman CL, Salamon ML, Blanchard GM, et al. Epidemiology of ankle arthritis: report of a consecutive series of 639 patients from a tertiary orthopaedic center. Iowa Orthop J 2005;25:44–6.
5. Adams SB, Demetracopoulos CA, Queen RM, et al. Early to Mid-Term Results of Fixed-Bearing Total Ankle Arthroplasty with a Modular Intramedullary Tibial Component. J Bone Joint Surg 2014;96(23):1983–9.
6. Valderrabano V, Horisberger M, Russell I, et al. Etiology of ankle osteoarthritis. Clin Orthop Relat Res 2009;467(7):1800–6.
7. Pierce Ebaugh M, Alford T, Kutzarov K, et al. Patient-Reported Outcomes of Primary Total Ankle Arthroplasty in Patients Aged <50 Years. Foot Ankle Orthop 2022;7(1). 24730114221082600.
8. Consul DW, Chu A, Langan TM, et al. Total Ankle Arthroplasty Survivorship, Complication, and Revision Rates in Patients Younger Than 55 Years. Foot Ankle Spec 2022;15(3):283–90.

9. Demetracopoulos CA, Adams SB, Queen RM, et al. Effect of Age on Outcomes in Total Ankle Arthroplasty. Foot Ankle Int 2015;36(8):871–80.
10. Usuelli FG, Maccario C, D'Ambrosi R, et al. Age-Related Outcome of Mobile-Bearing Total Ankle Replacement. Orthopedics 2017;40(3). https://doi.org/10.3928/01477447-20170327-05.
11. Coester LM, Saltzman CL, Leupold J, et al. Long-term results following ankle arthrodesis for post-traumatic arthritis. J Bone Joint Surg Am 2001;83(2):219–28.
12. Ling JS, Smyth NA, Fraser EJ, et al. Investigating the relationship between ankle arthrodesis and adjacent-joint arthritis in the hindfoot: a systematic review. J Bone Joint Surg Am 2015;97(6):513–20.
13. Dekker TJ, Hamid KS, Easley ME, et al. Ratio of Range of Motion of the Ankle and Surrounding Joints After Total Ankle Replacement: A Radiographic Cohort Study. J Bone Joint Surg 2017;99(7):576–82.
14. Glazebrook M, Daniels T, Younger A, et al. Comparison of Health-Related Quality of Life Between Patients with End-Stage Ankle and Hip Arthrosis. The Journal of Bone and Joint Surgery-American 2008;90(3):499–505.
15. Thomas R, Daniels TR, Parker K. Gait analysis and functional outcomes following ankle arthrodesis for isolated ankle arthritis. J Bone Joint Surg Am 2006;88(3):526–35.
16. Flavin R, Coleman SC, Tenenbaum S, et al. Comparison of gait after total ankle arthroplasty and ankle arthrodesis. Foot Ankle Int 2013;34(10):1340–8.
17. Pedowitz DI, Kane JM, Smith GM, et al. Total ankle arthroplasty versus ankle arthrodesis: a comparative analysis of arc of movement and functional outcomes. Bone Joint Lett J 2016;98-B(5):634–40.
18. SooHoo NF, Zingmond DS, Ko CY. Comparison of reoperation rates following ankle arthrodesis and total ankle arthroplasty. J Bone Joint Surg Am 2007;89(10):2143–9.
19. Ross BJ, Savage-Elliott I, Wu VJ, et al. Reoperation Rates Following Total Ankle Arthroplasty Versus Ankle Arthrodesis for Posttraumatic Indications. Foot Ankle Spec 2021. https://doi.org/10.1177/1938640021993630. 1938640021993630.
20. Ross BJ, Savage-Elliott I, Wu VJ, et al. Complications Following Total Ankle Arthroplasty Versus Ankle Arthrodesis for Primary Ankle Osteoarthritis. Foot Ankle Spec 2021. https://doi.org/10.1177/1938640020987741. 1938640020987741.
21. Goldberg AJ, Chowdhury K, Bordea E, et al. Total Ankle Replacement Versus Arthrodesis for End-Stage Ankle Osteoarthritis: A Randomized Controlled Trial. Ann Intern Med 2022;175(12):1648–57.
22. Stavrakis AI, SooHoo NF. Trends in Complication Rates Following Ankle Arthrodesis and Total Ankle Replacement. J Bone Joint Surg Am 2016;98(17):1453–8.
23. Younger ASE, Wing KJ, Glazebrook M, et al. Patient Expectation and Satisfaction as Measures of Operative Outcome in End-Stage Ankle Arthritis: A Prospective Cohort Study of Total Ankle Replacement Versus Ankle Fusion. Foot Ankle Int 2015;36(2):123 34.
24. Conlin C, Khan RM, Wilson I, et al. Living With Both a Total Ankle Replacement and an Ankle Fusion: A Qualitative Study From the Patients' Perspective. Foot Ankle Int 2021;42(9):1153–61.
25. Sangeorzan BJ, Ledoux WR, Shofer JB, et al. Comparing 4-Year Changes in Patient-Reported Outcomes Following Ankle Arthroplasty and Arthrodesis. J Bone Joint Surg 2021;103(10):869–78.
26. Haddad SL, Coetzee JC, Estok R, et al. Intermediate and long-term outcomes of total ankle arthroplasty and ankle arthrodesis. A systematic review of the literature. J Bone Joint Surg Am 2007;89(9):1899–905.

27. Zaidi R, Cro S, Gurusamy K, et al. The outcome of total ankle replacement: a systematic review and meta-analysis. Bone Joint Lett J 2013;95-B(11):1500–7.

28. Palanca A, Mann RA, Mann JA, et al. Scandinavian Total Ankle Replacement: 15-Year Follow-up. Foot Ankle Int 2018;39(2):135–42.

29. Bartel AFP, Roukis TS. Total Ankle Replacement Survival Rates Based on Kaplan-Meier Survival Analysis of National Joint Registry Data. Clin Podiatr Med Surg 2015;32(4):483–94.

30. Gougoulias N, Khanna A, Maffulli N. How successful are current ankle replacements?: a systematic review of the literature. Clin Orthop Relat Res 2010; 468(1):199–208.

31. Cody EA, Bejarano-Pineda L, Lachman JR, et al. Risk Factors for Failure of Total Ankle Arthroplasty With a Minimum Five Years of Follow-up. Foot Ankle Int 2019; 40(3):249–58.

32. Bernasconi A, Najefi AA, Goldberg AJ. Comparison of Mechanical Axis of the Limb Versus Anatomical Axis of the Tibia for Assessment of Tibiotalar Alignment in End-Stage Ankle Arthritis. Foot Ankle Int 2021;42(5):616–23.

33. Najefi AA, Malhotra K, Goldberg A. Mechanical and anatomical axis of the lower limb in total ankle arthroplasty. Foot 2020;44. 101666.

34. Najefi AA, Ghani Y, Goldberg A. Role of Rotation in Total Ankle Replacement. Foot Ankle Int 2019;40(12):1358–67.

35. Bracco P, Bellare A, Bistolfi A, et al. Ultra-High Molecular Weight Polyethylene: Influence of the Chemical, Physical and Mechanical Properties on the Wear Behavior. A Review. Materials 2017;10(7):791.

36. Losina E, Thornhill TS, Rome BN, et al. The Dramatic Increase in Total Knee Replacement Utilization Rates in the United States Cannot Be Fully Explained by Growth in Population Size and the Obesity Epidemic. The Journal of Bone and Joint Surgery-American 2012;94(3):201–7.

37. Saleh KJ, Dykes DC, Tweedie RL, et al. Functional outcome after total knee arthroplasty revision: a meta-analysis. J Arthroplasty 2002;17(8):967–77.

38. Ellington JK, Gupta S, Myerson MS. Management of failures of total ankle replacement with the agility total ankle arthroplasty. J Bone Joint Surg Am 2013;95(23):2112–8.

39. Hintermann B, Zwicky L, Knupp M, et al. HINTEGRA revision arthroplasty for failed total ankle prostheses. J Bone Joint Surg Am 2013;95(13):1166–74.

40. Williams JR, Wegner NJ, Sangeorzan BJ, et al. Intraoperative and perioperative complications during revision arthroplasty for salvage of a failed total ankle arthroplasty. Foot Ankle Int 2015;36(2):135–42.

41. Behrens SB, Irwin TA, Bemenderfer TB, et al. Clinical and Radiographic Outcomes of Revision Total Ankle Arthroplasty Using an Intramedullary-Referencing Implant. Foot Ankle Int 2020;41(12):1510–8.

42. Lachman JR, Ramos JA, Adams SB, et al. Patient-Reported Outcomes Before and After Primary and Revision Total Ankle Arthroplasty. Foot Ankle Int 2019; 40(1):34–41.

43. Schuberth JM, King CM, Jiang SF, et al. Takedown of Painful Ankle Arthrodesis to Total Ankle Arthroplasty: A Case Series of 77 Patients. J Foot Ankle Surg 2020; 59(3):535–40.

44. Lundeen AL, Raduan FC, Stone McGaver R, et al. Takedown of Ankle Fusions and Conversion to Total Ankle Replacements. Foot Ankle Int 2022;43(11):1402–9.

45. Pellegrini MJ, Schiff AP, Adams SB, et al. Conversion of Tibiotalar Arthrodesis to Total Ankle Arthroplasty. J Bone Joint Surg Am 2015;97(24):2004–13.

46. Kofoed H, Lundberg-Jensen A. Ankle arthroplasty in patients younger and older than 50 years: a prospective series with long-term follow-up. Foot Ankle Int 1999; 20(8):501–6.
47. Rodrigues-Pinto R, Muras J, Martín Oliva X, et al. Total ankle replacement in patients under the age of 50. Should the indications be revised? Foot Ankle Surg 2013;19(4):229–33.
48. Bayliss LE, Culliford D, Monk AP, et al. The effect of patient age at intervention on risk of implant revision after total replacement of the hip or knee: a population-based cohort study. Lancet 2017;389(10077):1424–30.
49. Ramaskandhan J, Rashid A, Kometa S, et al. Comparison of 5-Year Patient-Reported Outcomes (PROMs) of Total Ankle Replacement (TAR) to Total Knee Replacement (TKR) and Total Hip Replacement (THR). Foot Ankle Int 2020; 41(7):767–74.

Outcomes of Lateral Transfibular Approach for Total Ankle Replacement

Federico G. Usuelli, MD[a],*, Camilla Maccario, MD[a],
Cristian Indino, MD[a]

KEYWORDS

- Total ankle replacement • Lateral approach • Transfibular approach
- Fibula osteotomy • Trabecular metal • Ankle deformity • Ankle arthritis

KEY POINTS

- The main advantage of lateral approach is deformity correction, expanding surgical indications for total ankle replacement (TAR).
- The association of fibula osteotomy in combination with the use of a frame to achieve and stabilize deformity correction enhances the potential of correction on sagittal and rotational planes.
- Fibula osteotomy becomes now a tool of correction for coronal and rotational ankle deformities.
- TAR through lateral transfibular approach showed 97.7% survival rate at 5 years.

OVERVIEW

Since 1991 to 2010, data on total ankle replacement (TAR) reported a relative increase of 6.71-fold, along with a simultaneous 15.6% reduction of ankle arthrodesis (US data).[1]

TAR used to be a challenging treatment only for selected patients. Nowadays, TAR is gold standard treatment of ankle arthritis in high-volume centers with surgeons at the end of their learning curve.

TAR has been originally developed through an anterior approach. It allows direct visualization of the coronal alignment and an easy access to the medial-lateral edges of the joint.[2]

Although it is widely considered as the easiest and the most popular approach, anterior approach presents some limitations, especially when addressing sagittal malalignment deformities. These are not uncommon features in ankle arthritis.[3] According

[a] Ortopedia della Caviglia e del Piede, Humanitas San Pio X, Via Francesco Nava, 31, Milan 20159, Italy
* Corresponding author.
E-mail address: fusuelli@gmail.com

Foot Ankle Clin N Am 29 (2024) 69–80
https://doi.org/10.1016/j.fcl.2023.08.003
1083-7515/24/© 2023 Elsevier Inc. All rights reserved.

foot.theclinics.com

to the experience of the senior author, anterior talar shifting is much more frequent than posterior shifting and it is mainly related to 2 different patterns of pathology onset.

- Lateral ankle instability with rotational instability, resulting in a rotational deformity and anterior talar shifting (varus deformity)
- Posttraumatic posterior malleolus malreduction, resulting in syndesmotic pathologic condition and anterior talar shifting with a final equinus rigid deformity (equinus pseudovarus deformity) (**Fig. 1**).

Furthermore, recent implant designs are focused on bone-preserving cut and low-volume implants, especially for talar component. With an anterior approach, this may imply the choice of a more proximal tibial cut in order to allow joint preparation and implants positioning.[4] Poor-quality bone and pegs fixation could be reasons for tibial osteolysis.[4,5]

In 2012, lateral transfibular approach was reintroduced as part of a new concept of direct vision on the center of rotation of ankle joint, with bone-preserving and curved-shaped cuts and implants (TM Ankle, Zimmer Biomet, Warsaw, Indiana).

It was originally advertised as a safer approach in terms of wound healing issues but further data did not confirm this assumption.[6]

The main advantage of lateral approach, claimed by their users, is deformity correction, expanding surgical indications for TAR.

The major complaint against this procedure is syndesmotic joint disruption that may lead to loosening of correction and valgus failure.

Anyway, data at 5 years confirm this is a safe procedure even in case of preoperative valgus deformity.[7,8] Of course, longer follow-up are needed.

LATERAL TRANSFIBULAR APPROACH

Lateral transfibular approach for TAR was originally proposed for St Georg in 1973 and subsequently for the ESKA (ESKA, Germany) in 1990.[9,10] Both of them were not successful procedures and were abandoned.

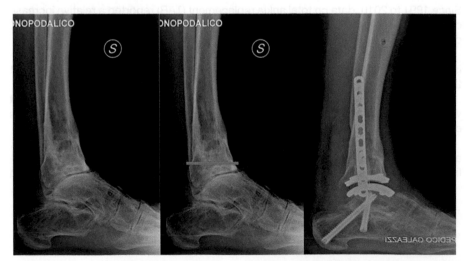

Fig. 1. Anterior shifting related to posterior malleolus malreduction. Lateral preop, lateral preop theoretic plan for tibial cut with an anterior approach, lateral approach allows shifting correction and curved preserving cut on both surfaces (tibia and talus).

In the recent years, the successful development of ankle replacement with anterior approach brought to a better understanding of frequent reasons for failures: technical mistakes, tibial subsidence and periarticular cysts, and infections.

These 3 topics may explain a new interest toward lateral approach.

Technical Mistake and Power of Correction

Lateral approach allows a direct vision on the center of rotation, resulting in a more accurate sagittal deformity correction.[6,11–15]

Furthermore, the association of fibula osteotomy in combination with the use of a frame to achieve and stabilize deformity correction (before articular preparation) enhances the potential of correction on both sagittal and rotational planes.[11]

Anyway, as any surgical complex procedure, the results are affected by surgeon learning curve.

Maccario and colleagues (2021) described learning curve for TAR with transfibular approach for a surgeon with a previous experience in TAR.[16] They reported on 114 cases followed-up for 24 to 61 months: surgical time decreased with the curve stabilizing after the 16th patient; visual analogue scale (VAS), American Orthopedic Foot and Ankle Society Score (AOFAS), and Short Form - 12 Mental Component Score (SF-12 MCS) scores stabilized after 21, 13, and 16, respectively; sagittal talar alignment and tibial coronal alignment stabilized at 18 and 15 patients; minor complication rates curve stabilized after the 39th patient; no significant learning curve was found for ankle range of motion and tibial sagittal alignment.

Regardless of approaches and implants, efficient training program should be considered an ethical duty for companies producing TARs. However, stakeholders (hospital, ambulatory surgery centers, and health-care associations) involved in ankle arthritis treatment should be sensitive to this topic. High-volume reference centers have a deep role that still needs to be designed.

Finally, the combination of direct vision on the center of rotation and curved bony cut allows the surgeon to proximally or distally shift the new center of rotation (ankle off-set).[17] This has an influence on implant stiffness (too distal center of rotation positioning) and implant instability (too proximal center of rotation positioning).

Tibial Subsidence and Periarticular Cysts

Reasons for cyst developing are still under debate. It has been shown a strong correlation with tibial component fixation (stem should be avoided[4]; **Fig. 2**).

Some authors correlate it with mobile-bearing but there is no consensus.[18]

Tibial radiolucency and consequent possible subsidence should be considered as a different topic. It could be related to several factors but one of the most relevant is tibial quality bone. Allowing curved cut for both surfaces (tibia and talar ones), transfibular lateral approach technique preserves tibial anterior cortex, which has been described as the highest quality bone area for axial load and implant osteointegration.[19]

Finally, both tibia and talar components rely on trabecular metal for bone-surface fixation (metal-back). Its powerful osteointegration properties have already been showed in other anatomic districts.[20,21]

These features may help to explain the reduced risk of subsidence reported in literature with lateral transfibular approach implants.[8] No periarticular cysts have been reported.[8]

Infections

There is no significant difference comparing anterior and lateral approach for infections and would healing issues.[6]

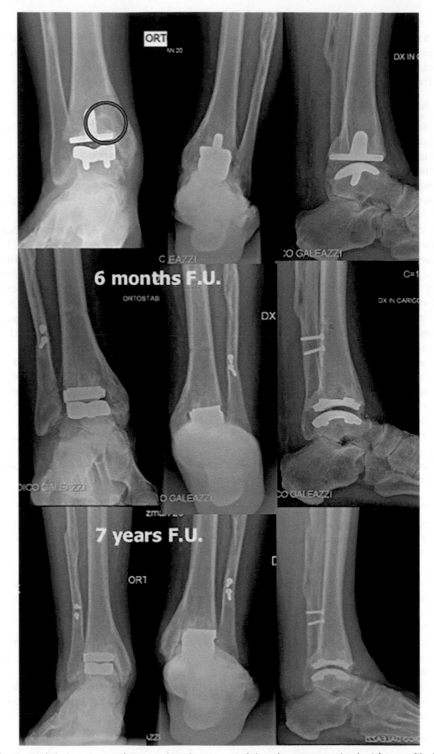

Fig. 2. Mobile bearing and stem-related cysts: painful replacement revised with transfibular approach. Final follow-up at 7 years.

Anyway, wound healing issues may end up in skin failure problems. If that is the case, for anterior approach, it means implant exposure and failure.

For lateral approach, it means fibular fixation exposure. This is a less risky condition, which can be addressed with hardware removal.

Disadvantages have also been reported with lateral approach: increased operative time, fibular osteotomy with a risk of delayed union or nonunion, the potential for symptoms related to the fibular implant.[12,14,15,22]

Osteotomy Modification (FARG Osteotomy): Fibula Osteotomy A, a Tool of Correction

The original surgical technique describes a short oblique fibular osteotomy to access the tibiotalar joint.[23]

It was approximately 2 cm long, starting at the proximal part of the lateral aspect of the fibula, extending distally and medially, and ending 1 to 1.5 cm proximal to the tibiotalar joint with plate fixation at the end of the whole procedure.[24]

The main disadvantage is hardware bulkiness (anatomic plate) and possible symptoms related to the fibular plate and wound issues requiring hardware removal.[6,12,22] A further disadvantage is a lower power of correction for this osteotomy, not allowing fibula lengthening either shortening.

Our group introduced a modification of this osteotomy with longer fibular osteotomy (Foot and Ankle Reconstruction Group: "FARG" Osteotomy).

It starts 6 to 7 cm proximal to the tibiotalar joint line, extended from posterosuperior to anteroinferior and ends 2 cm proximal to the joint line.[11] It allows fibula shortening/lengthening and abduction/adduction.

FARG Fibula osteotomy becomes now a tool of correction for coronal and rotational ankle deformities.

Moreover, this kind of osteotomy can be fixed with 3 parallel free cortex screws (3.5 mm screws) in most of the cases, showing a decrease rate of wound complications and no need for hardware removal procedure.[11]

Additional Medial Approach, When?

Medial gutter debridement may be necessary in case of deltoid calcification or heterotopic calcification between medial malleolus and talar medial wall. These are the cases where an additional medial approach is recommended. According to senior author experience, it is more likely to happen in preoperative severe varus deformity (less than 5% of the cases).

A secondary medial approach has been also described to address medial pain after TAR, as a revision surgery.[25]

Medial pain is not an infrequent complaint regardless of the approach and implant choice. According the experience of the senior author, it is unlikely for this procedure to be completely successful. In case of medial pain, conservative treatment is recommended for the first postop year. In case of persistent medial pain, it is advisable to look for a rotational malalignment and triceps power unbalance.

Implant and Surgical Technique

The TM Ankle system was approved by the US Food and Drug Administration in 2012. This prosthesis consists of a 2-component semiconstrained fixed-bearing implant. An alignment coordinate system and a milling device guide the bone resections and facilitate addressing both varus, valgus, rotational, and sagittal deformities.[24] The alignment stand is a rigid coordinate system to base the bony resections and it enables correction of sagittal and coronal deformities, theoretically improving the reliability of the positioning of the implants.[24]

The implant novelty includes unique shape of joint congruency, curved rather than flat cuts on bone, highly cross-linked fixed polyethylene bearing, and the use of tantalum metal for the bone surface fixation.[16] The tantalum metal is heated in chlorine gas with vitreous carbon, resulting in material knowns as trabecular metal.[26]

OUTCOMES

Two nondesigner prospective studies recently reported results on transfibular TAR.

The first one reported 97.7% survival rate at 5 years on 86 patients. The cohort of patients included posttraumatic arthritis in 88.8%, rheumatoid arthritis in 5.6%, and degenerative joint disease secondary to congenital clubfoot in 2.2%.[8]

No evidence of periprosthetic cysts was reported. No evidence of subsidence but asymptomatic radiolucency was found in 9.3% of the cases. About 8.1% of the patients received lateral hardware removal and 1.2% of the patients received syndesmotic screw removal. About 2.3% reported wound healing issues, successfully treated. About 2.3% experienced deep infections with implant failures.[8]

The second one is an international nondesigner multicenter prospective cohort study on 121 patients with 97.35% survival and 92.5% satisfaction rates at 3 years.[27]

About 35% of the patients were affected by rheumatoid arthritis. Infection rate was 0.83%, and lateral hardware removal rate was 6.6%.[27]

Interestingly, both of the studies report no fibular nonunion.

Tiusanen and colleagues reported diverging but still promising results on 104 patients at 43 months follow-up.[28]

He claimed a 38% of reoperation rate, mostly related to wound healing issues and requiring hardware removal.[28] Higher hardware removal rate may be related to the use of anatomic plates for fibular fixation. Anatomic plates definitely provide more stability but determine higher mechanical stress for lateral soft tissue.

We support the adoption of 3-screw fixation technique if possible (FARG osteotomy). When it is not, we recommend the use of one-third tubular plates.[11]

In 2018, Barg and colleagues, reported good outcomes but tibia radiolucency in 35% of the cases as an early report.[22]

The lower rate described in the previous prospective article (9.3%) may be related to the cementless technique coupled with trabecular metal and early weight-bearing protocols, described by the authors.[8]

Coronal Deformity Outcomes

Historically, deformity used to be considered an absolute contraindication for TAR.

Evolution of both surgical technique and implants widened these borders.

Literature proved that deformity is not a contraindication for TAR.[7,29,30] Furthermore, the final result is more affected by postoperative alignment than preoperative deformity.

Our group proved the reliability of this technique for both varus and valgus deformity[7,29] (Fig 3).

Especially in valgus deformities, which are usually considered the most challenging ones, Piga and colleagues reported no significant difference between neutral and valgus ankle (above 10°) with no loosing of correction at 2 years on a total sample of 228 cases.[7]

Senior author recommends to avoid underestimating the role of bony accessory procedures in order to achieve the overall alignment of the lower limb (Fig. 4).

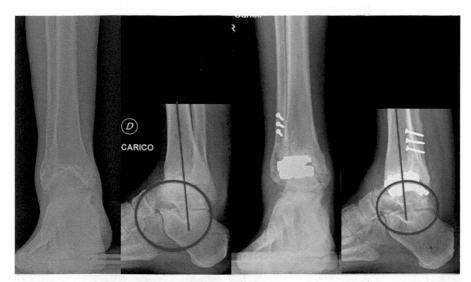

Fig. 3. Varus arthritic ankle: varus is a rotational, multiplanar deformity, affected by anterior shifting. Lateral transfibular approach allows direct vision on the center of rotation reliable anterior talar shifting correction. Preop and 3-year postop radiographs.

The frame is a useful intraoperative tool to correct any intra-articular deformities and to correlate these corrections to the lower limb alignment. It is not a device to correct extra-articular deformity. Preoperative planning with weight-bearing imaging will preoperatively disclose the need of additional bony procedure.[31]

Special attention should be paid to the soft tissue management, especially in valgus deformity. Although there is no evidence, authors suggest to consider vacuum assisted closure (VAC) therapy as postop medication in valgus cases with poor soft tissue envelope.

Sagittal Deformity: a Paradigm Shifting

Lateral transfibular approach is a paradigm shifting that disclosed interest on different prospective only occasionally mentioned before.

Coronal deformity is a 3 dimensions deformity, with a concomitant sagittal and rotational deformity.

Some patterns of coronal deformity express a significant sagittal deformity that need to be addressed.[3]

For instance, varus deformity related to ankle instability has a common pattern of evolution in anterior talar shifting. Joint instability anteriorly drives talus. This results in an anterior talar shifting and anterior tibial slope. The key to a successful treatment is joint realignment on both coronal and sagittal plane, addressing the anterior shifting.

A second frequent pattern for developing anterior-shifting is related to posterior malleolar fracture malreduction. Posterior shifted malleolus and pathologic syndesmotic joint act together as a lever arm, pushing talus anteriorly and sticking the ankle in rigid equinus deformity. These patients usually present a clinical equinus pseudovarus feature, that evolve in valgus once the equinus is intraoperatively addressed. Sagittal anatomic repositioning is a critical point for a long-term and stable correction.

The direct vision on the center of rotation of the joint allows a better vision and evaluation of this parameter in combination with an efficient coronal plane correction.

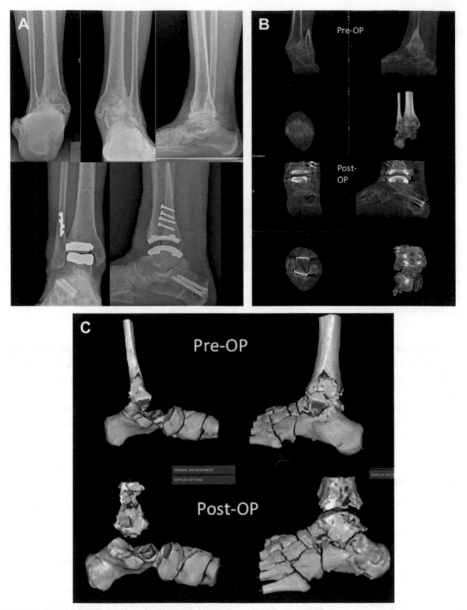

Fig. 4. (*A*) Valgus arthritic ankle with Progressive Collapsing foot: weight-bearing preop and postop radiographs: no loosing of correction at 2 years follow-up. (*B*) Same previous valgus case studied with WB CT scan. Preop coronal view shows lateral calcaneo-fibular impinge-ment. Postop coronal view shows stable improvement of lateral calcaneo-fibular impinge-ment obtained thorough ankle alignment (transfibular ankle replacement) and medial calcaneal displacement. (*C*) Preop and postop syndesmotic stress analyzed with semiauto-matic measuring system (BoneLogic–Disior, Englewood, CO, USA). Distance Mapping tool was used. It measures gap between articular surfaces. It is an indirect measure of joint over-load (physiologic green to pathologic red). In this case, it shows a reduced distal stress around syndesmotic joint after the surgery. Lateral approach is a tool to improve deformity correction and it does not negatively affect syndesmotic function.

Missing Fibula: "Milanese Technique"

The presence of an intact distal fibula is reported as a prerequisite when considering TAR, and its lack is usually considered a contraindication.[32]

In case of missing fibula for a previous infection, trauma, severe fibula shortening for previous ankle fracture, lateral approach represents an easy access to the pathologic ankle.

The fibular reconstruction Milanese technique is an alternative surgical technique to reconstruct an absent or insufficient lateral malleolus in the setting of a TAR.[33]

According to this technique, proximal residual fibula can be rotated laterally and distally with the aim to keep muscular insertions and vascularity. It is eventually fixed to tibia with minimum three 4.5 lag screws, restoring the proper distal fibula length (**Fig. 5**).

A series of 15 cases have been recently described, with no complications directly related to this lateral malleolus reconstruction.[33]

Considering the lack of data, it is still a surgical technique that could be considered in limited cases as a complex lower limb salvage procedure.

Fast-Track Rehabilitation and Fibula Osteotomy. Are They Compatible?

Enhanced recovery protocols were popularized in hip and knee replacements with proven advantages for patients.[34,35]

Early weight-bearing exposure and early walking exercise are also possible for a select group of patients with TAR and lateral transfibular approach.

We recently described a Fast Track Score in order to identify patients eligible to immediate weight-bearing postop management.[36] The Key Performance Indicators mentioned in this Score are body mass index, state of anxiety or depression, functional preoperative status, preop equinus deformity, preop coronal alignment, surgical time, surgical accessory procedures, and bone quality.

Considering the posttraumatic cause in most of the cases, patients affected by ankle arthritis are 7 to 11 years younger than patients with end-stage hip and knee arthritis at surgery time.[37]

This may be the reasons for higher expectations in patients affected by ankle arthritis. Fast-track protocol, when possible, plays a key role to respond to these goals.

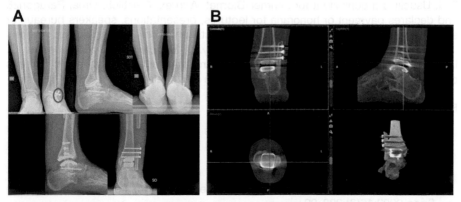

Fig. 5. (A) Milanese Technique–Missing Fibula: posttraumatic ankle infection previously treated with Cement Spacer. Preop with cement spacer and first weight-bearing postop with TAR and Milanese technique at 3 months. (B) WB CT scan 4 years after surgery showing physiologic alignment.

SUMMARY

Even if TAR through a lateral transfibular approach has been introduced as a safer approach in terms of wound healing issues, still no significant difference comparing anterior and lateral approach was detected with the numbers available. However, the main advantage of this technique is proved to be the correction of deformities through action and optimal view on coronal, sagittal, and rotational issues, conjugated with the possibility of correction of fibular length discrepancy. It showed reliable outcomes at 5 years follow-up with a survival rate of 97.7%.

CLINICS CARE POINTS

- In 2012, lateral transfibular approach was reintroduced as part of a new concept of direct vision on the center of rotation of ankle joint, with bone-preserving and curved-shaped cuts and implants.
- As any surgical complex procedure, the results are influenced by surgeon's learning curve.
- Trabecular metal improves osteointegration and reduces the risks of osteolysis.
- There is no significant difference comparing anterior and lateral approach for infections and would healing issues but the main advantage is deformity control and fibular length correction.
- A survival rate of 97.7% at 5 years on 86 patients has been reported.

FUNDING

F.G. Usuelli is a consultant for Zimmer-Biomet, Arthrex, BRM, Episurf, Geistlich, Lima, Paragon28, Planmed. He declares payment or honoraria for lectures, presentations, speakers bureaus or educational events, and payment for expert testimony from Zimmer Biomet, Arthrex, Geistlich. He received royalties from Paragon28. Zimmer Biomet supported educational grant in his institution.

DISCLOSURE

F.G. Usuelli is a consultant for Zimmer-Biomet, Arthrex, Geistlich, Lima, Paragon28 and declares payment or honoraria for lectures, presentations, speakers bureaus or educational events, and payment for expert testimony from Zimmer Biomet, Arthrex, Geistlich all of which are unrelated to this study. C. Maccario has no disclosures. C. Indino declares payment or honoraria for lectures, presentations, speakers bureaus or educational events from Arthrex, all of which are unrelated to this study.

REFERENCES

1. Pugely AJ, Lu X, Amendola A, et al. Trends in the use of total ankle replacement and ankle arthrodesis in the United States Medicare population. Foot Ankle Int 2014;35(3):207–15.
2. Kim J, Gagne OJ, Rajan L, et al. Clinical Outcomes of the Lateral Trabecular Metal Total Ankle Replacement at a 5-Year Minimum Follow-up. Foot Ankle Spec 2023;16(3):288–99.
3. Usuelli FG, Manzi L, Brusaferri G, et al. Sagittal tibiotalar translation and clinical outcomes in mobile and fixed-bearing total ankle replacement. Foot Ankle Surg 2017;23(2):95–101.

4. Yu J, Zhang C, Chen WM, et al. Finite-element analysis of the influence of tibial implant fixation design of total ankle replacement on bone-implant interfacial biomechanical performance. J Orthop Surg (Hong Kong) 2020;28(3). 2309499020966125.

5. Kim S, Jang J, Choi J-H, et al. Volume and Distribution of Periprosthetic Bone Cysts in the Distal Tibia and Talus before Early Revision of Total Ankle Arthroplasty. Appl Sci 2021;11(16):7242.

6. Usuelli FG, Indino C, Maccario C, et al. Infections in primary total ankle replacement: Anterior approach versus lateral transfibular approach. Foot Ankle Surg 2019;25(1):19–23.

7. Piga C, Maccario C, D'Ambrosi R, et al. Total Ankle Arthroplasty With Valgus Deformity. Foot Ankle Int 2021;42(7):867–76.

8. Maccario C, Paoli T, Romano F, et al. Transfibular total ankle arthroplasty : a new reliable procedure at five-year follow-up. Bone Joint Lett J 2022;104-B(4):472–8.

9. Engelbrecht E. Ankle-joint endoprosthesis model "St. George". Z Orthop Ihre Grenzgeb 1975;113(4):546–8.

10. Rudigier J, Grundei H, Menzinger F. Prosthetic replacement of the ankle in post-traumatic arthrosis 10-yearex perience with the cementless ESKA ankle prosthesis. Eur J Trauma 2001;27(2):66–74.

11. Usuelli FG, Indino C, Maccario C, et al. A Modification of the Fibular Osteotomy for Total Ankle Replacement Through the Lateral Transfibular Approach. J Bone Joint Surg Am 2019;101(22):2026–35.

12. Tan EW, Maccario C, Talusan PG, et al. Early complications and secondary procedures in transfibular total ankle replacement. Foot Ankle Int 2016;37(8):835–41. Epub 2016 Apr 20.

13. Goetz JE, Rungprai C, Tennant JN, et al. Variable Volumes of Resected Bone Resulting From Different Total Ankle Arthroplasty Systems. Foot Ankle Int 2016; 37(8):898–904.

14. Usuelli FG, Maccario C, Indino C, et al. Tibial slope in total ankle arthroplasty: Anterior or lateral approach. Foot Ankle Surg 2017;23(2):84–8.

15. Usuelli FG, Maccario C, Granata F, et al. Clinical and Radiological Outcomes of Transfibular Total Ankle Arthroplasty. Foot Ankle Int 2019;40(1):24–33.

16. Maccario C, Tan EW, Di Silvestri CA, et al. Learning curve assessment for total ankle replacement using the transfibular approach. Foot Ankle Surg 2021; 27(2):129–37.

17. Harnroongroj T, Hummel A, Ellis SJ, et al. Assessing the Ankle Joint Line Level Before and After Total Ankle Arthroplasty With the "Joint Line Height Ratio". Foot Ankle Orthop 2019;4(4). 2473011419884359.

18. Lachman J, Taylor M, Cody E, et al. A Comparison of Cyst Formation and Management in Mobile-Bearing and Fixed-Bearing Total Ankle Arthroplasty. Foot Ankle Orthop 2019;4(2). 2473011419S00005.

19. Easley ME, Vertullo CJ, et al. Total Ankle Arthroplasty. J Am Acad Orthop Surg 2002;10(3):157–67.

20. López-Torres II, Sanz-Ruíz P, Sánchez-Pérez C, et al. Clinical and radiological outcomes of trabecular metal systems and antiprotrusion cages in acetabular revision surgery with severe defects: a comparative study. Int Orthop 2018; 42(8):1811–8.

21. Fernandez-Fairen M, Hernández-Vaquero D, Murcia A, et al. Trabecular metal in total knee arthroplasty associated with higher knee scores: a randomized controlled trial. Clin Orthop Relat Res 2013;471(11):3543–53.

22. Barg A, Bettin CC, Burstein AH, et al. Early clinical and radiographic outcomes of trabecular metal total ankle replacement using a transfibular approach. J Bone Joint Surg Am 2018;100(6):505–15.
23. Usuelli FG, D'Ambrosi R, Manzi L, et al. Treatment of Ankle Osteoarthritis with Total Ankle Replacement Through a Lateral Transfibular Approach. J Vis Exp 2018; 131:56396.
24. Usuelli FG, Indino C, Maccario C, et al. Total ankle replacement through a lateral approach: surgical tips. SICOT J 2016;2:38.
25. Kim BS, Choi WJ, Kim J, et al. Residual pain due to soft-tissue impingement after uncomplicated total ankle replacement. Bone Joint Lett J 2013;95-B(3):378–83.
26. Kormi S, Kohonen I, Koivu H, et al. Low Rate of Peri-implant Osteolysis in Trabecular Metal Total Ankle Replacement on Short- to Midterm Follow-up. Foot Ankle Int 2021;42(11):1431–8.
27. D'Ambrosi R, Tiusanen HT, Ellington JK, et al. Fixed-Bearing Trabecular Metal Total Ankle Arthroplasty Using the Transfibular Approach for End-Stage Ankle Osteoarthritis: An International Non-Designer Multicenter Prospective Cohort Study. JB JS Open Access 2022;7(3):e2100143.
28. Tiusanen H, Kormi S, Kohonen I, et al. Results of Trabecular-Metal Total Ankle Arthroplasties With Transfibular Approach. Foot Ankle Int 2020;41(4):411–8.
29. Usuelli FG, Di Silvestri CA, D'Ambrosi R, et al. Total ankle replacement: is preoperative varus deformity a predictor of poor survival rate and clinical and radiological outcomes? Int Orthop 2019;43(1):243–9.
30. de Keijzer DR, Joling BSH, Sierevelt IN, et al. Influence of Preoperative Tibiotalar Alignment in the Coronal Plane on the Survival of Total Ankle Replacement: A Systematic Review. Foot Ankle Int 2020;41(2):160–9.
31. VandeLune C, Barbachan Mansur NS, Iehl C, et al. Deformity Correction in Ankle Osteoarthritis Using a Lateral Trans-Fibular Total Ankle Replacement: A Weight-Bearing CT Assessment. Iowa Orthop J 2022;42(2):36–46.
32. Bonasia DE, Dettoni F, Femino JE, et al. Total ankle replacement: why, when and how? Iowa Orthop J 2010;30:119–30.
33. Usuelli FG, de Cesar Netto C, Maccario C, et al. Reconstruction of a missing or insufficient distal fibula in the setting of a total ankle replacement: The Milanese technique. Foot Ankle Surg 2022;28(2):186–92.
34. Hirschmann MT, Kort N, Kopf S, et al. Fast track and outpatient surgery in total knee arthroplasty: beneficial for patients, doctors and hospitals. Knee Surg Sports Traumatol Arthrosc 2017;25(9):2657–8.
35. Wainwright TW, Gill M, McDonald DA, et al. Consensus statement for perioperative care in total hip replacement and total knee replacement surgery: Enhanced Recovery After Surgery (ERAS®) Society recommendations. Acta Orthop 2020; 91(1):3–19.
36. Usuelli FG, Paoli T, Indino C, et al. Fast-Track for Total Ankle Replacement: A Novel Enhanced Recovery Protocol for Select Patients. Foot Ankle Int 2023; 44(2):148–58.
37. Herrera-Pérez M, Valderrabano V, Godoy-Santos AL, et al. Ankle osteoarthritis: comprehensive review and treatment algorithm proposal. EFORT Open Rev 2022;7(7):448–59.

Outcomes of Total Ankle Replacement with Preoperative Varus Deformity

Laurian J.M. van Es, MD[a,b], Daniel Haverkamp, MD, PhD[b],
Niek C. van Dijk, MD, PhD[c,d,e,f], Laurens W. van der Plaat, MD[g],*

KEYWORDS

- Varus deformity • Preoperative alignment • Total ankle arthroplasty
- Total ankle replacement • Medial malleolar osteotomy • Deltoid release

KEY POINTS

- Varus deformity can be structurally corrected during/after TAR through correctly applied ancillary procedures.
- Increasing varus deformity appears to negatively influence TAR survival.
- Clinical scores are similar for TAR in neutral and varus ankles.
- Heterogeneity of results impairs drawing scientifically sound conclusions regarding controversies of TAR in varus-deformed ankles.

INTRODUCTION

Recent data estimate the 10-year survival of total ankle replacement (TAR) ranging from 69% to 85%.[1–3] Though hardly close to the results of hip arthroplasties and knee arthroplasties,[4–6] TAR survival is reported to improve with more modern designs.[7] Furthermore, focus shifting toward patient mobility and quality of life seems to contribute to the popularity of TAR.[8] Patient characteristics currently considered risk factors for TAR failure are high load cycles, lower age at implantation, high body mass index (BMI) or high activity level, (uncontrolled) diabetes, peripheral vascular disease, and poor baseline Ankle

[a] Department of Orthopedic Surgery, Tergooi MC, Van Riebeeckweg 212, 1213 XZ Hilversum, the Netherlands; [b] Department of Orthopedic Surgery, Xpert Clinics, SCORE Foundation, Specialized Center of Orthopedic Research and Education, Laarderhoogtweg 12, 1101AE, Amsterdam, the Netherlands; [c] Department of Orthopedic Surgery, Amsterdam UMC location AMC, Posthus 22660, 1100 DD Amsterdam Zuidoost, the Netherlands; [d] Head of Ankle Unit, FIFA Medical Centre of Excellence Ripoll-DePrado Sport Clinic Madrid, Spain; [e] Head of Ankle Unit, FIFA Medical Centre of Excellence Clínica do Dragão Porto, Portugal; [f] Casa di Cura San Rossore, Viale delle Cascine, 152/f, 56122 Pisa Italy; [g] Department of Traumatology and Orthopedic Surgery, St.-Antonius-Hospital Kleve, Klinik für Unfallchirurgie und Orthopädie, Albersallee 5-7, Kleve 47533, Germany
[*] Corresponding author.
E-mail address: Laurens.vanderplaat@kkle.de

Foot Ankle Clin N Am 29 (2024) 81–96
https://doi.org/10.1016/j.fcl.2023.09.007

Osteoarthritis Scale scores.[9–11] Historically, coronal plane deformities of greater than 10° to 15° have been deemed contraindications.[12,13] However, recent studies report satisfactory results in TAR with severe preoperative varus or valgus angles.[14–17]

Deformity correction is highly important[18–22] as incomplete correction induces postoperative edge-loading, which can result in malleolar fractures, ligament instability, progressive deformity, polyethylene wear, pain, osteolysis, component loosening, or clinical failure.[13,16,22–24]

DEFORMITY TYPES
Coronal Plane Deformities

The majority (55%) of osteoarthritic ankles have a varus deformity (when defined as the angle between the tibial shaft and the talar dome <90°), while only 8% will present with a valgus deformity (when defined as the angle between the tibial shaft and the talar dome >99°).[25] Varus deformity of the ankle indicates a decrease of the tibiotalar angle, which has been shown to average 92.4° ± 3.1° on radiographs in adults[26] (**Fig. 1**). Several studies report the outcome of TAR in coronally deformed ankles, but the definition of deformity used varies (**Table 1**).

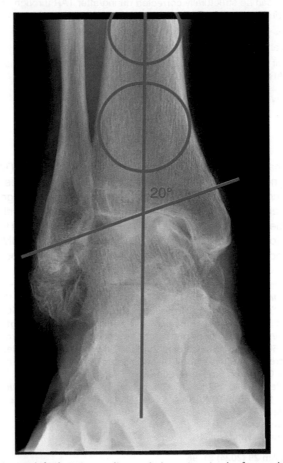

Fig. 1. Preoperative weight-bearing radiograph (mortise view) of an ankle with an incongruent varus deformity of approximately 20°.

Table 1
Results of studies on total ankle replacement in preoperatively varus-deformed ankles

Authors, Year	Prosthesis Design	N	Average FU (mth)	Definition of Varus (°)	Preoperative Ti-Ta Angle (°)	Standard Additional Procedure(s)	Additional Procedures[a]	Complications	Non-revision sec. Surgery	Revisions	AOFAS
Haskell et al,[24] 2004	Star	25	23	>10	16.5	Deltoid release	+	+	12% (3/25)	4% (1/25)	-
Henricson, et al,[57] 2007	Star, BP, AES	55	50	>5	9.6[b]	None	+	+	18% (10/55)	31% (17/55)	-
Kim, et al,[35] 2009	Hintegra	23	27	>10	17.1	Deltoid release	78% (18/23)	9% (2/23)[c]	-	9% (2/23)	83
Wood, et al,[70] 2010	Mobility	33	43	-	-	None	+	+	+	3% (1/33)	+
Shock, et al,[41] 2011	Salto Talaris, INBONE	26[d]	17	>5	16.8	Deltoid sleeve	38% (10/26)	-	-	4% (1/26)	-
Reddy, et al,[67] 2011	STAR	23	41	>10	18.1	None	+	+	+	+	-
Trincat et al,[42] 2012	AES, Salto, New-Jersey	15	36	>10	6.1	None	>100% (30/15)	40% (6/15)	40% (6/15)	13% (2/15)	72
Trajkovski, et al,[16] 2013	Hintegra, Mobility, Star	36	37	>10	19.9	None	81% (29/36)	42% (15/36)	33% (12/36)	8% (3/36)	81
Sproule et al,[71] 2013	Mobility	26	40	-	-	None	+	+	+	8% (2/26)	+
Queen, et al,[68] 2013	Salto Talaris, INBONE	27	24	5-15	9.2	None	>100% (38/27)	30% (8/27)	22% (6/27)	4% (1/27)	+
Sung, et al,[15] 2014	Hintegra, Mobility	24	25	>20	25.7	Medial periosteal release	71% (17/24)	25% (6/24)	-	4% (1/24)	83
Joo, et al,[66] 2017	Hintegra	35 35 Tot: 70	46 50 Tot: 48	5-15 >15	9.4 20.0	None	57% (20/35) 60% (21/35)	34% (12/35) 54% (19/35) Tot: 44%	- -	3% (1/35) 3% (1/35) Tot: 3% (2/70)	92 92

(continued on next page)

Table 1
(continued)

Authors, Year	Prosthesis Design	N	Average FU (mth)	Definition of Varus (°)	Preoperative Ti-Ta Angle (°)	Standard Additional Procedure(s)	Additional Procedures[a]	Complications	Non-revision sec. Surgery	Revisions	AOFAS
Cottom et al,[62] 2018	Star	16	36	>5	12.2	AL & partial deltoid release	100% (16/16)	-	-	-	88
Krishnapillai, et al,[72] 2019	BP	17	109	>4	-	None	+	+	+	12% (2/17)	-
Allport et al,[51] 2021	Mobility	60	56	>10	18.1	None	48% (29/60)	+	23% (14/60)	8% (5/60)	-
Umbel, et al,[17] 2022	Infinity, INBONE II	12, 6, 1, Tot: 19	37	6–10, 11–15, >15	7.6, 11.5, 16.3	None	>100% (24/12), >100% (25/6), >100% (3/1), Tot: 100%	30% (4/12), 30% (2/6), 100% (1/1), Tot: 37% (7/19)[c]	30% (4/12), 15% (1/6), 0%, Tot: 26% (5/19)	0%, 17% (1/6), 100% (1/1), Tot: 11% (2/19)	-, -, -, -
Van Es, et al,[50] 2022	CCI	61	83	>5	-	None	+	+	43% (26/61)[e]	25% (15/61)[||]	-
Boble et al,[60] 2022	Salto, Salto Talaris	31, 26, Tot: 57[d] 29	26, 31	5–15, >15	9.2, 19.7	Circular release & posterior capsulectomy	>100% (77/31), >100% (80/26), Tot: 28% (16/57)	35% (11/31), 19% (5/26), Tot: 28% (16/57)	19% (6/31), 4% (1/26), Tot: 12% (7/57)	10% (3/31), 8% (2/26), Tot: 9% (5/57)	80, 81
Yamashita et al,[65] 2022	TNK	16	29	>10	13.9	None	63% (10/16)	44% (7/16)	-	13% (2/16)	-
Van der Plaat, et al,[43] 2022	BP, CCI, AAA	95[d]	71	-	12.4	Medial malleolar osteotomy	33% (31/95)	44% (42/95)[c]	22% (21/95)	29% (28/95)	-

This table is an updated extension of previous searches.[43,49]

Abbreviations: AL, achilles tendon lengthening; AOFAS, American Orthopedic Foot & Ankle Society hindfoot score; FU, Follow-up; mth, months; sec., secondary; Ti-Ta, Tibiotalar; Tot, total; +, described but not quantifiable; -, not described.

[a] In case of greater than 100%, only the total number of additional procedures could be extracted from the article instead of the % of ankles receiving additional procedures.

[b] Clinical measurement.

[c] Only revisions treated surgically.

[d] Studies solely reporting on TAR in varus-deformed ankles.

[e] Data extracted from own database.

The cause of ankle malalignment can either be extra-articular (proximal or distal) or intra-articular.[20,27] Examples of proximal extra-articular causes of ankles deformity are malunions of the tibia or osteoarthritis of the knee. Distally, hindfoot and forefoot deformities may play a part in the deformity of the ankle joint.[20] Intra-articular causes can be bone erosion, tibial plafond malunion, talar necrosis, ectopic ossifications in the joint gutters, lateral ligament laxity leading to instability, or deltoid ligament contracture.[28]

Intra-articular deformities can be further divided into congruent (meaning the talus and tibia plafond appear parallel on radiographs) and incongruent (meaning deviating talar alignment compared to the tibia dome).[24]

Sagittal Plane Deformities

Though not the scope of this article, it is equally vital to acknowledge sagittal plane deformities such as equinus position or post-traumatic distal tibial recurvatum. The remainder of the current article will focus solely on TAR with varus deformity.

DEFORMITY CORRECTION

The surgical procedure(s) applied for correcting the varus deformity depend on the type of deformity observed. Several (slightly differing) treatment algorithms have been developed to address this issue.[27,29–32]

The first decision is whether correction can be obtained during TAR implantation or a staged procedure is indicated. Staged procedures should be performed in case of extra-articular deformities proximal to the ankle joint (eg, varus osteoarthritis of the knee joint, tibial shaft malunion, genu varum).[32,33] In case of supramalleolar varus deformity, however, both 1-stage and 2-stage corrections have been advocated.[27,33,34]

Furthermore, a 2-stage procedure might be considered in following situations: an arthritic subtalar joint that requires arthrodesis; a rigid subtalar joint with medial translation of the calcaneus upon the talus that requires arthrodesis; gross lateral ligament instability with associated severe foot pathology; and prior attempts at cavovarus foot correction with insufficient correction.[33]

The surgical strategies used during TAR to obtain correction of the varus deformity generally start with adequate removal of osteophytes and gutter debridement. The (adjusted) bone cuts for the prosthetic components may be sufficient for solitary medial bone erosion or in case of minimal lateral laxity[28]; however, it is unknown to which degree. Good outcome has been reported in cases up to 16° of preoperative congruent varus.[35] In case of remaining tibiotalar incongruence, ancillary procedures are performed.

Medial Release

Mainly 3 surgical techniques are described to release medial tightness.[21,28–31,34,36–41] First, a (deep) deltoid ligament release[16,28] at the medial talar border. Alternatively, a complete periosteal flap dissection of the deltoid ligament at its origin at the medial malleolus (deltoid ligament sleeve)[28]. Working from anterior to posterior, the superficial and deep ligaments are released, whereafter, the surgeon can consider additionally cleaving the posterior tendon sheet.[28] Lastly, a medial malleolar osteotomy (MMO) can be performed.[15,28,42] The osteotomy (by oscillating saw or osteotome) is made craniomedially at a 45° angle a few millimeters distal to the tibial plafond to prevent weakening the medial tibial plafond thereby risking varus collapse of the tibial component.[37] Some variants of this procedure are described regarding the timing of the osteotomy (before or after the bone cuts[43]) **(Fig. 2)**, and the use of osteosynthetic fixation or bone-grafts[27,44] **(Fig. 3)**.

Adjuncts to the medial release by means of tendinous procedures like tibialis anterior or posterior (split) transfer[32,45] have been described.

Lateral Reconstruction

The presence of lateral structure laxity can be resolved through capsule plication, lateral ligament reconstruction (like [modified] Bröstrom,[46] or use of [prosthetic] graft[47]), fibular shortening, or peroneal tendon (split) transfers to the lateral cuneiform bone[45] or onto peroneus brevis tendon.[35]

DEFORMITY DISTALLY TO THE TIBIOTALAR JOINT AFTER TAR IS TREATED, DEPENDING ON THE CAUSE

Persistent hindfoot varus can be treated using a lateralizing calcaneus osteotomy or calcaneal wedge osteotomy.[34] Forefoot supination can be treated using a dorsiflexion osteotomy at the basis of the first metatarsal or dorsiflexion arthrodesis of the first tarsometatarsal joint.[34] A medialized, shortened Achilles tendon might contribute to the deformity and can be treated using a tenotomy or gastric slide. As the anteromedial fibers of the Achilles tendon originate from the soleus muscle and the anterior, posterior, and lateral fibers originate from the gastrocnemius muscle,[48] it could be theorized that a tenotomy would lead to a stronger correction when compared to a gastric slide.

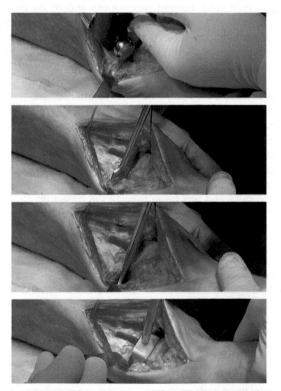

Fig. 2. Procedure of medial malleolar osteotomy (MMO). The series of photos depict: i. performing osteotomy by oscillating saw (in this picture as an horizontal cut), ii: finalizing osteotomy by osteotome, iii: presentation of the MMO, and iv: fitting the trial components and testing for collateral stability.

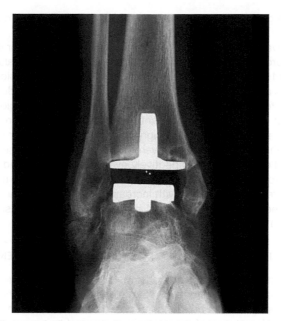

Fig. 3. Postoperative weight-bearing radiograph (mortise view) of total ankle replacement (TAR) with MMO without osteosynthetic fixation.

Unfortunately, due to absence of studies directly comparing these various procedures, it is still unclear which (combination) of procedures would produce the best results in each patient.

RESULTS OF TAR IN ANKLES WITH PREOPERATIVE NEUTRAL VERSUS NON-NEUTRAL ALIGNMENT

The last systematic review regarding the influence of preoperative coronal plane deformities on the survival of TAR, published in 2020, described revisions per 100 component years (/100cpy).[49] Seventeen studies (13 retrospective, 3 prospective, and 1 randomized trial), comprising 1692 TARs with a mean follow-up of 4.4 years, were included. The ankles comprised 711 neutral, 545 varus, and 332 valgus alignments. Another 104 ankles were unspecified. The definition of varus was greater than 5° deviation in 6 and greater than 10° in 10 studies. One study lacked a definition. The neutrally aligned ankles showed 1.6 revisions/100cpy and required additional procedures in 41% of the cases. The varus group showed 1.7 revisions/100cpy and additional procedures in 92% of the cases. The valgus group showed 2.5 revisions/100cpy and additional procedures in 65% of the cases. The authors concluded that preoperative varus alignment showed comparable implant survival, and valgus alignment demonstrated negative influence compared to neutral alignment.

Since then, new studies reporting revision rates in neutrally versus non-neutrally aligned ankles have been published.[50,51] Van Es and colleagues analyzed the ceramic coated implant (CCI) mobile-bearing prosthesis at a mean 6.9 years of follow-up and found lower survival in the deformed (>5°) group. When subdivided into varus, valgus, and neutral, the significance faded.[50] Allport and colleagues, reporting on the Mobility mobile-bearing prosthesis, found identical survival after 56 months in the neutral and deformed (>10°) group. However, more additional procedures were performed in the deformed group.[51]

Two studies evaluated preoperative alignment as a risk factor for revision (both using HINTEGRA prosthesis),[52,53] of which Richter and colleagues evaluated the 10-year revision rates of 1006 TAR. There was no increased chance of revision in preoperative varus and valgus ankles compared to neutral ankles. However, ankles with a preoperative major hindfoot deformity (medial distal tibial angle and tibiotalar angle <83° or >95°) showed a statistically significant Hazard ratio of 2.5 for revision compared to neutrally aligned ankles, while the significance disappeared for minor deformities versus neutral ankles. Valgus ankles were more likely to be revised than varus ankles.[52] Zafar and colleagues retrospectively evaluated 322 TAR and found a reduced risk (mean Hazard ratio 0.95) per degree of increased preoperative medial talar angle, suggesting that revisions increase with increasing preoperative varus angles.[53] Likewise, a decreased postoperative medial distal tibial angle (increased varus position of the prosthesis) increased the risk of revision.

RESULTS OF TAR IN ANKLES WITH PREOPERATIVE VARUS ALIGNMENT

An updated selection (eg, studies comprising <15 TARs were excluded) of the studies included in the previously mentioned systematic review regarding the results of TAR in varus-deformed ankles[49] can be found in **Table 1**. It consists of a heterogenic pool of data, including various types of procedure(s) performed to correct the deformity. The data are further confounded by different prostheses (including abandoned implants, eg, ankle evolutive system (AES),[54,55] CCI,[50] Mobility[7,56]), bearing types, deformity severity, registered parameters, and follow-up.

Summarizing the results of these studies despite their heterogeneity leads to the following conclusions.

Survival/Revision Rates

Revision rates vary from 3% to 31%, with follow-up varying from 17 to 109 months. Three studies showed revision rates of 25% to 30% of the cases.[43,50,57] Van Es and colleagues reported 25% revisions, resulting in a 10-year survival of 48%, which the authors blamed on the prosthesis design (CCI).[50] Henricson and colleagues reported a 31% revision rate at 50 months average follow-up, with the majority of revisions being performed at short-term follow-up due to technical error or instability.[57] Van der Plaat and colleagues reported a 29% revision rate at 71 months of average follow-up in ankles treated with the combination of TAR and MMO.[43]

Non-revision Secondary Surgery

Non-revision reoperation rates are reported in less than 50% of the studies in **Table 1**. They range from 15% to 43%, with follow-up varying from 37 to 83 months, which is globally similar to non-revision reoperation rates in regular TAR cohorts.[58,59]

Ancillary Procedures

Nearly all studies in **Table 1** reported the necessity of performing additional (often more than one[15,41,42,45,60–65]) procedures to obtain a plantigrade foot during TAR implantation.[16,41,49,51,61,63,64,66] As the level of deformity increases, more additional procedures are required per case.[14,67] Additional procedures are needed significantly more in varus ankles, compared to neutrally aligned ankles.[16,51,66] Interestingly, surgical duration has been reported to not differ substantially between deformed and non-deformed ankles.[63]

Complications

According to the latest systematic review, complication rates in varus and neutrally aligned ankles are similar at 24%.[49] However, the authors' updated literature search reveals higher average complication rates of 25% to 46%, with follow-up varying from 24 to 71 months. One study reported outlying results with a complication rate of 9% in 23 TAR at 27 months average follow-up.[35] However, only major complications necessitating reoperations were reported.

Clinical Scores

Globally speaking, no significant differences in either increase of, or score at final follow-up, between the various alignment groups were reported regarding clinical scores (eg, AOFAS), patient-reported outcome measures (PROM), or pain scores.[15,16,35,60,63–66,68] Interestingly, 1 study reported better mental health scores at final follow-up in the varus ankles compared to the neutral ankles and similar findings for the domains "function," "social," and "health" of the Self-Administered Foot Evaluation Questionnaire were reported in another study.[16,65] Similar findings have been reported before.[69–72]

DISCUSSION

According to the latest systematic review, revision rates of TAR in varus-deformed ankles are similar to those in neutral ankles.[49] However, recent research hints at decreasing survival with increasing deformity.[51–53] Likewise, complications are supposedly similar in deformed and neutral ankles at 24% according to this systematic review,[49] although the authors' updated search revealed multiple studies with around 40% complication rates. The number of non-revision reoperations are comparable in neutral and deformed cohorts, as are clinical scores, but the number of ancillary procedures needed to obtain a plantigrade foot is substantially greater in deformed ankles.

As stated before, these conclusions are based on heterogeneous data sets with multiple confounding factors, 1 of these being the type of prosthesis used (fixed vs mobile bearing). Most articles stemming from the United States report on fixed-bearing prostheses, as up until now the Scandinavian total ankle replacement (STAR)prosthesis is the only mobile-bearing device with Food and Drug Administration approval,[73] while in Europe, mobile-bearing devices are generally the primarily used implants. Recently, the hindfoot position has been shown to be static with a mobile-bearing TAR while changing over time after implantation of a fixed-bearing TAR.[74] This might indicate that optimal alignment of the prosthetic components is even more critical in fixed-bearing implants than in mobile-bearing implants.

A second confounding factor is found in the potentially performed ancillary procedure(s). These are, generally speaking, chosen on the basis of the nature of the deformity and intraoperative observations and sometimes deviating from available algorithms (eg, tibialis anterior transfer[45] and synthetic graft lateral ankle stabilization[47]). An example is the choice between medial soft tissue (deltoid) release and MMO.

Studies with specific results of TAR with MMO are scarce. Doets and colleagues first described the technique in 2008, reporting neutral postoperative ankle alignment in all 15 patients with a mean preoperative varus deformity of 15° (BP and CCI prosthesis). However, in addition to 1 revision, 3 ankles needed secondary surgery to correct persistent hindfoot varus.[37]

Van der Plaat and colleagues reported 29% revisions and 44% reoperations at an average follow-up of 5.9 years in a series of 95 TARs (Triple A [AAA], Buechel-Pappas

[BP], and CCI) with MMO with an average preoperative varus deformity of 12°. However, postoperative radiological alignment was not described.[43]

Lastly, Hirao and colleagues found no differences in clinical scores and PROMs in 27 TAR (FINE) with MMO compared to 30 regular TARs in patients with rheumatoid arthritis at 8 years of average follow-up. All osteotomies united without internal fixation (15% took longer than 12 weeks), lateral malleolar fractures occurred in 19%, but revision rates were not provided.[44]

Studies with specific results of TAR with deltoid release are likewise scarce. Kim and colleagues treated 23 varus ankles with TAR (Hintegra) combined with a medial release. The clinical and radiological results at an average follow-up of 27 months were similar to those of the neutral ankles.[35] Two ankles in the varus group were revised. Shock and colleagues reported correction of deformity in 26 varus ankles by means of TAR (Salto Talaris and Inbone) with complete deltoid sleeve release after an average follow-up of 17 months, with 1 needing revision.[41] Lastly, Cottom and colleagues reported maintenance of deformity correction in 16 varus ankles treated with TAR (STAR) with (partial) deltoid release, with a follow-up of 36 months.[62]

Obviously, due to confounding factors like types of prostheses, bearing types, and duration of follow-up, drawing conclusions on MMO versus deltoid release is currently impossible.

A third confounding factor is the type of deformity. Congruent and incongruent varus deformities have been studied in a few studies with approximately 3 years of average follow-up and sample sizes of about 25 patients. Haskell and colleagues found that incongruent joints were 10 times more likely to develop progressive edge-loading than congruent joints, and all reoperations were performed on ankles with preoperative incongruence.[24] Trincat and colleagues reported more ancillary procedures, more complications, and more (non)revision reoperations in the varus-incongruent group.[42] Contrary to these findings, Kim and colleagues found comparable results between congruent and incongruent ankles regarding complications, revisions, and functional outcome.[35]

CONCLUSION

Current literature hints at increasing complications and revision rates in TAR of varus-deformed ankles when compared to regular TAR, especially with increasing deformity. The needed number of ancillary procedures increases with increasing deformity, however, non-revision surgery and clinical scores are comparable to those reported for regular TAR. Obtaining a stable prosthesis with a neutrally-aligned hindfoot at the end of the procedure still appears of paramount importance. Drawing scientifically sound conclusions regarding some of the controversies of TAR in varus deformity is currently impossible due to the heterogeneity of data.

FUTURE DIRECTIONS
Prediction of Needed Ancillary Procedures (Surgical Planning)

Last years, Lintz and colleagues have been studying 3-dimensional (3D) foot and ankle biomechanics using weight-bearing CT.[75] One measurement, in particular, is the Foot and Ankle Offset (FAO), a software calculation representing the offset between the hindfoot-forefoot midline and the center of the talar dome, normalized for foot length. It describes the hindfoot alignment, with a mean FAO of 2.3%, −11.6%, and 11.4% in patients with a clinically neutral, varus, and valgus hindfoot (respectively) and has been shown to have excellent interobserver reliability.[75,76] It is reported that an increased risk of lateral and medial pathologies of the foot and ankle exist at an FAO of < −1.6% and greater than 2.7%, respectively.[77]

The FAO was analyzed to predict the necessity of intraoperative additional proced-ures during TAR.[78] The FAO showed a significant, positive correlation with the number of ancillary osseous procedures, not with total and/or soft tissue procedures. Out of all specific procedures performed, deltoid ligament release and medial column procedures showed a significant correlation with an R^2 value of 0.7. The number of osseous realign-ment procedures was significantly higher in valgus malalignment when compared to varus malalignment. Especially, medial column realignment procedures were 6.3 times more needed in the valgus versus the varus group. The authors suggest that the FAO can be a reliable tool in assessing preoperative deformity and surgical planning.

To solve the heterogeneity of data on TAR in varus or even better, TAR in general, an international consensus group (ideally including people involved in national joint reg-istries) could define guidelines for registration of patient characteristics (eg, cause of arthritis, comorbidities, smoking, activity level). An example being the international consensus meeting on surgical site and periprosthetic joint infection.[79] Likewise, (the method of measuring) alignment should be quantified. Consensus on the use of PROMs and a uniform definition of "revision" is needed. Complications should be uni-formly registered (for which several classifications have been proposed[80,81]) as strat-ification of risk to prosthetic survival is needed.[82] Furthermore, as both native and prosthetic varus and valgus knees have been shown to exhibit different kinematics,[83] and this might also be the case in the (prosthetic) ankle joint, separation of results of varus and valgus ankles appears warranted.

SUMMARY

When correctly applying ancillary procedures before, during, or after TAR, correction of varus deformity can be maintained over time, resulting in similar clinical scores as those obtained with TAR in non-deformed ankles. Complications and revision rates appear to increase with increasing varus deformity, but current literature does not sup-port the afore-mentioned historical threshold above which TAR is contraindicated as heterogeneity of data precludes strict conclusions.

CLINICS CARE POINTS

- Varus deformity can be structurally corrected during/after TAR through correctly applied ancillary procedures.
- Increasing varus deformity appears to negatively influence TAR survival.
- Clinical scores are similar for TAR in neutral and varus ankles.
- Heterogeneity of results impairs drawing scientifically sound conclusions regarding controversies of TAR in varus-deformed ankles.

DISCLOSURE

The authors have nothing to disclose.

REFERENCES

1. Henricson A, Nilsson J, Carlsson A. 10-year survival of total ankle arthroplasties: a report on 780 cases from the Swedish Ankle Register. Acta orthopedic 2011; 82(6):655–9.

2. Onggo JR, Nambiar M, Phan K, et al. Outcome after total ankle arthroplasty with a minimum of five years follow-up: A systematic review and meta-analysis. Foot Ankle Surg 2020;26(5):556–63.
3. Association NZO. The New Zealand Joint Registry, twenty-two year report. 2020.
4. van der Plaat LW, Hoornenborg D, Sierevelt IN, et al. Ten-year revision rates of contemporary total ankle arthroplasties equal 22%. A meta-analysis. Foot Ankle Surg 2021. https://doi.org/10.1016/j.fas.2021.05.014.
5. Evans JT, Evans JP, Walker RW, et al. How long does a hip replacement last? A systematic review and meta-analysis of case series and national registry reports with more than 15 years of follow-up. Lancet (London, England) 2019; 393(10172):647–54.
6. Evans JT, Walker RW, Evans JP, et al. How long does a knee replacement last? A systematic review and meta-analysis of case series and national registry reports with more than 15 years of follow-up. Lancet (London, England) 2019; 393(10172):655–63.
7. Undén A, Jehpsson L, Kamrad I, et al. Better implant survival with modern ankle prosthetic designs: 1,226 total ankle prostheses followed for up to 20 years in the Swedish Ankle Registry. Acta Orthop 2020;91(2):191–6.
8. Fanelli D, Mercurio M, Castioni D, et al. End-stage ankle osteoarthritis: arthroplasty offers better quality of life than arthrodesis with similar complication and re-operation rates—an updated meta-analysis of comparative studies. Int Orthop 2021. https://doi.org/10.1007/s00264-021-05053-x.
9. Escudero MI, Le V, Barahona M, et al. Total ankle arthroplasty survival and risk factors for failure. Foot Ankle Int 2019;40(9):997–1006.
10. van der Plaat LW, Haverkamp D. Patient selection for total ankle arthroplasty. Orthop Res Rev 2017;9:63–73.
11. Hermus JPS, van Kuijk SMJ, Spekenbrink-Spooren A, et al. Risk factors for total ankle arthroplasty failure: A Dutch Arthroplasty Register study. Foot Ankle Surg 2022;28(7):883–6.
12. Doets HC, Brand R, Nelissen RG. Total ankle arthroplasty in inflammatory joint disease with use of two mobile-bearing designs. J Bone Joint Surgery 2006; 88(6):1272–84.
13. Wood PL, Deakin S. Total ankle replacement. The results in 200 ankles. J Bone Joint Surgery 2003;85(3):334–41.
14. Lee GW, Lee KB. Outcomes of total ankle arthroplasty in ankles with >20° of coronal plane deformity. J Bone Joint Surgery 2019;101(24):2203–11.
15. Sung KS, Ahn J, Lee KH, et al. Short-term results of total ankle arthroplasty for end-stage ankle arthritis with severe varus deformity. Foot Ankle Int 2014;35(3): 225–31.
16. Trajkovski T, Pinsker E, Cadden A, et al. Outcomes of ankle arthroplasty with preoperative coronal-plane varus deformity of 10° or greater. J Bone Joint Surgery 2013;95(15):1382–8.
17. Umbel BD, Hockman T, Myers D, et al. Accuracy of CT-derived patient-specific instrumentation for total ankle arthroplasty: the impact of the severity of preoperative varus ankle deformity. Foot Ankle Spec 2022. 19386400211068262.
18. Conti SF, Wong YS. Complications of total ankle replacement. Clin Orthop Relat Res 2001;(391):105–14.
19. de Asla RJ, Ellis S, Overley B, et al. Total ankle arthroplasty in the setting of valgus deformity. Foot Ankle Spec 2014;7(5):398–402.
20. Greisberg J, Hansen ST Jr. Ankle replacement: management of associated deformities. Foot Ankle Clin 2002;7(4):721–36, vi.

21. Stamatis ED, Myerson MS. How to avoid specific complications of total ankle replacement. Foot Ankle Clin 2002;7(4):765–89.
22. Wood PL, Sutton C, Mishra V, et al. A randomised, controlled trial of two mobile-bearing total ankle replacements. J Bone and Joint Surgery 2009;91(1):69–74.
23. Sugimoto K, Samoto N, Takakura Y, et al. Varus tilt of the tibial plafond as a factor in chronic ligament instability of the ankle. Foot Ankle Int 1997;18(7):402–5.
24. Haskell A, Mann RA. Ankle arthroplasty with preoperative coronal plane deformity: short-term results. Clin Orthop Relat Res 2004;(424):98–103.
25. Valderrabano V, Horisberger M, Russell I, et al. Etiology of ankle osteoarthritis. Clin Orthop Relat Res 2009;467(7):1800–6.
26. Knupp M, Ledermann H, Magerkurth O, et al. The surgical tibiotalar angle: a radiologic study. Foot Ankle Int 2005;26(9):713–6.
27. Adams SB, Steele JR, Demetracopoulos CA, et al. Results of tibia and fibula osteotomies performed concomitant to total ankle replacement. Foot Ankle Int 2020; 41(3):259–66.
28. Coetzee J, Rippstein P. Total ankle replacement in deformity. The atlas of ankle replacements. World Scientific 2021;345–68.
29. Choi WJ, Kim BS, Lee JW. Preoperative planning and surgical technique: how do I balance my ankle? Foot Ankle Int 2012;33(3):244–9.
30. Knupp M, Bolliger L, Barg A, et al. [Total ankle replacement for varus deformity]. Orthopä 2011;40(11):964–70.
31. Ryssman DB, Myerson MS. Total ankle arthroplasty: management of varus deformity at the ankle. Foot Ankle Int 2012;33(4):347–54.
32. Daniels TR. Surgical technique for total ankle arthroplasty in ankles with preoperative coronal plane varus deformity of 10° or greater. JBJS Essential Surgical Techniques 2014;3(4):e22.
33. Steginsky B, Haddad SL. Two-stage varus correction. Foot Ankle Clin 2019;24(2): 281–304.
34. Ryssman D, Myerson MS. Surgical strategies: the management of varus ankle deformity with joint replacement. Foot Ankle Int 2011;32(2):217–24.
35. Kim BS, Choi WJ, Kim YS, et al. Total ankle replacement in moderate to severe varus deformity of the ankle. J Bone Joint Surgery 2009;91(9):1183–90.
36. Barg A, Pagenstert GI, Leumann AG, et al. Treatment of the arthritic valgus ankle. Foot Ankle Clin 2012;17(4):647–63.
37. Doets HC, van der Plaat LW, Klein JP. Medial malleolar osteotomy for the correction of varus deformity during total ankle arthroplasty: results in 15 ankles. Foot Ankle Int 2008;29(2):171–7.
38. Orthner E. Total ankle arthroplasty in varus instability–a new method of correction. Fuß Sprungg. 2011;9:96–101.
39. Roukis TS. Modified evans peroneus brevis lateral ankle stabilization for balancing varus ankle contracture during total ankle replacement. J foot and ankle surgery 2013;52(6):789–92.
40. Schuberth JM, Christensen JC, Seidenstricker CL. Total ankle replacement with severe valgus deformity: technique and surgical strategy. J Foot and Ankle Surgery 2017;56(3):618–27.
41. Shock RP, Christensen JC, Schuberth JM. Total ankle replacement in the varus ankle. J Foot and Ankle Surgery 2011;50(1):5–10.
42. Trincat S, Kouyoumdjian P, Asencio G. Total ankle arthroplasty and coronal plane deformities. Orthopaedics & Traumatology, Surgery & Research 2012;98(1): 75–84.

43. van der Plaat LW, Doets HC, van Dijk CN, et al. Medial malleolar osteotomy for the correction of tibiotalar varus deformity during total ankle arthroplasty: Results in 95 ankles. Foot 2022;52:101905.

44. Hirao M, Hashimoto J, Ebina K, et al. Radiographic effects observed in the coronal view after medial malleolar osteotomy at total ankle arthroplasty in rheumatoid arthritis cases. J Orthopaedic Science 2020;25(6):1072–8.

45. Hamel J. Early results after tibialis anterior tendon transfer for severe varus in total ankle replacement. Foot Ankle Int 2012;33(7):553–9.

46. Karlsson J, Bergsten T, Lansinger O, et al. Reconstruction of the lateral ligaments of the ankle for chronic lateral instability. J Bone and Joint Surgery 1988;70(4):581–8.

47. Rushing CJ, McKenna BJ, Berlet GC. Lateral instability in total ankle arthroplasty: a comparison between the brostrom-gould and anatomic lateral ankle stabilization (ATLAS). Foot Ankle Spec 2021. 19386400211041897.

48. Szaro P, Witkowski G, Smigielski R, et al. Fascicles of the adult human Achilles tendon - an anatomical study. Annals of anatomy = Anatomischer Anzeiger 2009;191(6):586–93.

49. de Keijzer DR, Joling BSH, Sierevelt IN, et al. Influence of preoperative tibiotalar alignment in the coronal plane on the survival of total ankle replacement: a systematic review. Foot Ankle Int 2020;41(2):160–9.

50. van Es LJM, van der Plaat LW, Sierevelt IN, et al. Long-term follow-up of 254 ceramic coated implant (CCI) evolution total ankle replacements. Foot Ankle Int 2022;43(10):1285–94.

51. Allport J, Ramaskandhan J, Alkhreisat M, et al. Patient-reported outcome measures and radiological outcomes in mobile-bearing total ankle arthroplasty with varus or valgus deformity. Foot Ankle Int 2021;42(2):176–82.

52. Richter D, Krähenbühl N, Susdorf R, et al. What are the indications for implant revision in three-component total ankle arthroplasty? Clin Orthop Relat Res 2021;479(3):601–9.

53. Zafar MJ, Kallemose T, Benyahia M, et al. 12-year survival analysis of 322 Hintegra total ankle arthroplasties from an independent center. Acta Orthop 2020; 91(4):444–9.

54. Koivu H, Kohonen I, Mattila K, et al. Medium to long-term results of 130 Ankle Evolutive System total ankle replacements-Inferior survival due to peri-implant osteolysis. Foot Ankle Surg 2017;23(2):108–15.

55. Kokkonen A, Ikävalko M, Tiihonen R, et al. High rate of osteolytic lesions in medium-term followup after the AES total ankle replacement. Foot Ankle Int 2011;32(2):168–75.

56. Raglan M, Machin JT, Cro S, et al. Total ankle replacement: comparison of the outcomes of STAR and Mobility. Acta Orthop Belg 2020;86(1):109–14.

57. Henricson A, Ågren P-H. Secondary surgery after total ankle replacement: The influence of preoperative hindfoot alignment. Foot Ankle Surg 2007;13(1):41–4.

58. Stadler C, Luger M, Stevoska S, et al. High reoperation rate in mobile-bearing total ankle arthroplasty in young patients. Medicina (Kaunas, Lithuania) 2022;58(2).

59. Gaugler M, Krähenbühl N, Barg A, et al. Effect of age on outcome and revision in total ankle arthroplasty. The bone & joint journal 2020;102-b(7):925–32.

60. Boble M, Le Nail LR, Brilhault J. Impact of preoperative varus on ankle replacement survival. Orthopaedics & traumatology, surgery & research : OTSR 2022; 108(7):103390.

61. Lee GW, Wang SH, Lee KB. Comparison of intermediate to long-term outcomes of total ankle arthroplasty in ankles with preoperative varus, valgus, and neutral alignment. J Bone and Joint Surgery 2018;100(10):835–42.
62. Cottom JM, Plemmons BS, Douthett SM. A critical radiographic analysis of coronal plane deformity correction using a 3-piece mobile bearing ankle joint replacement: a retrospective study of 25 patients. J Foot Ankle Surgery 2018;57(6):1161–6.
63. Usuelli FG, Di Silvestri CA, D'Ambrosi R, et al. Total ankle replacement: is preoperative varus deformity a predictor of poor survival rate and clinical and radiological outcomes? Int Orthop 2019;43(1):243–9.
64. Johnson MD, Shofer JB, Hansen ST Jr, et al. The impact of coronal plane deformity on ankle arthrodesis and arthroplasty. Foot Ankle Int 2021;42(10):1294–302.
65. Yamashita T, Nagai K, Kanzaki N, et al. Short-term clinical outcomes following total ankle arthroplasty without concomitant osteotomy in ankles with severe preoperative varus deformity: comparison to ankles with preoperative neutral alignment. J Am Podiatric Medical Association 2022;112(6).
66. Joo SD, Lee KB. Comparison of the outcome of total ankle arthroplasty for osteoarthritis with moderate and severe varus malalignment and that with neutral alignment. Bone & Joint Journal 2017;99-b(10):1335–42.
67. Reddy SC, Mann JA, Mann RA, et al. Correction of moderate to severe coronal plane deformity with the STAR ankle prosthesis. Foot Ankle Int 2011;32(7):659–64.
68. Queen RM, Adams SB Jr, Viens NA, et al. Differences in outcomes following total ankle replacement in patients with neutral alignment compared with tibiotalar joint malalignment. J Bone Joint Surgery 2013;95(21):1927–34.
69. Hobson SA, Karantana A, Dhar S. Total ankle replacement in patients with significant pre-operative deformity of the hindfoot. J Bone Joint Surg 2009;91(4):481–6.
70. Wood PL, Karski MT, Watmough P. Total ankle replacement: the results of 100 mobility total ankle replacements. J Bone Joint Surgery 2010;92(7):958–62.
71. Sproule J, Chin T, Amin A, et al. Clinical and radiographic outcomes of the mobility total ankle arthroplasty system: early results from a prospective multicenter study. Foot Ankle Int 2013;34(4):491–7.
72. Krishnapillai S, Joling B, Sierevelt IN, et al. Long-term follow-up results of buechel-pappas ankle arthroplasty. Foot Ankle Int 2019;40(5):553–61.
73. Noori NB, Ouyang JY, Noori M, et al. A review study on total ankle replacement. Appl Sci 2023;13(1):535.
74. Usuelli FG, Maccario C, Indino C, et al. Evaluation of hindfoot alignment after fixed- and mobile-bearing total ankle prostheses. Foot Ankle Int 2020;41(3):286–93.
75. Lintz F, Welck M, Bernasconi A, et al. 3D Biometrics for hindfoot alignment using weightbearing CT. Foot Ankle Int 2017;38(6):684–9.
76. Zhang JZ, Lintz F, Bernasconi A, et al. 3D Biometrics for hindfoot alignment using weightbearing computed tomography. Foot Ankle Int 2019;40(6):720–6.
77. Lintz F, Ricard C, Mehdi N, et al. Hindfoot alignment assessment by the foot-ankle offset: a diagnostic study. Arch Orthop Trauma Surg 2022. https://doi.org/10.1007/s00402-022-04440-2.
78. de Cesar Netto C, Day J, Godoy-Santos AL, et al. The use of three-dimensional biometric foot and ankle offset to predict additional realignment procedures in total ankle replacement. Foot Ankle Surg 2022;28(7):1029–34.
79. Parvizi J, Gehrke T, Chen AF. Proceedings of the International consensus on periprosthetic joint infection. Bone & Joint Journal. 2013;95-b(11):1450–2.

80. Gadd RJ, Barwick TW, Paling E, et al. Assessment of a three-grade classification of complications in total ankle replacement. Foot Ankle Int 2014;35(5):434–7.
81. Glazebrook MA, Arsenault K, Dunbar M. Evidence-based classification of complications in total ankle arthroplasty. Foot Ankle Int 2009;30(10):945–9.
82. Knabel M, Cook JJ, Basile P, et al. Risk stratification for revision surgery following total ankle replacement. J Foot and Ankle Surgery 2022;61(3):551–6.
83. Baier C, Benditz A, Koeck F, et al. Different kinematics of knees with varus and valgus deformities. J Knee Surgery 2018;31(3):264–9.

Bilateral Total Ankle Arthroplasty

Amanda N. Fletcher, MD, MS*

KEYWORDS

- Bilateral • Total ankle replacement • Total ankle arthroplasty • Staged
- Simultaneous • Ankle arthritis

KEY POINTS

- Patients with bilateral ankle arthritis have higher rates of primary and secondary/inflammatory arthritis and a more debilitating condition than those with unilateral pathology.
- The utilization and indications for total ankle arthroplasty (TAA) have expanded during the past decade, including patients undergoing bilateral TAA.
- Bilateral TAA is a treatment option for patients with bilateral end-stage ankle arthritis who have failed conservative treatment modalities.
- The potential benefits of the single anesthesia event, shorter rehabilitation period, and reduced cost must be weighed with the possible perioperative risk.

INTRODUCTION

The utilization and indications for total ankle arthroplasty (TAA) have expanded during the past decade, including patients undergoing bilateral TAA. Bilateral TAA is a treatment option for patients with bilateral end-stage ankle arthritis who have failed conservative treatment modalities. This may include patients with osteoarthritis, inflammatory arthritis, or bilateral lower extremity trauma. The decision to perform single-stage bilateral TAA (1 operative event) versus 2-stage TAA (2 operative events) remains a source of controversy in the ankle arthroplasty as well as hip and knee arthroplasty literature. The potential benefits of the single anesthesia event, shorter rehabilitation period, and reduced cost must be weighed with the possible perioperative risk.

Terminology

The terminology surrounding bilateral arthroplasty is inconsistent and may be confusing when reading and critically evaluating the arthroplasty literature. Different terms of reference include simultaneous, staged, sequential, and so forth. When

Ortho Carolina Foot & Ankle Institute, Charlotte, NC, USA
* 2001 Vail Avenue, Suite 200B, Charlotte, NC 28207-1222.
E-mail address: ancfletcher@gmail.com

Foot Ankle Clin N Am 29 (2024) 97–109
https://doi.org/10.1016/j.fcl.2023.08.004
1083-7515/24/© 2023 Elsevier Inc. All rights reserved.
foot.theclinics.com

assessing the literature, it is important to determine the setting of the bilateral procedures.

1. Single-stage bilateral TAA: occurs in one operative setting
   a. One-surgeon/operative team performing the arthroplasty surgeries sequentially or one after the other (ie, right followed by left).
      i. Most bilateral arthroplasty studies perform the surgeries in this manner. This method is commonly referred to as "simultaneous" given the bilateral joints are replaced in the same operative setting.
   b. Two-surgeons/operative teams performing the arthroplasty surgeries simultaneously or in parallel.
      i. This may also be referred to as "simultaneous" but is much less common than the 1-surgeon method.
2. Two-stage (staged) bilateral TAA: occurs in 2 operative settings
   • Some may also refer to this as "sequential."
   • It is important to evaluate if these procedures were truly "staged" and discussed preoperatively or if the contralateral extremity became symptomatic at a later time point.

For the simplicity of this article and consistency with previous literature, the surgeries will be referred to as simultaneous (single-stage) or staged (2-stage) bilateral TAA. Simultaneous will refer to a single-stage, 1-surgeon operative team unless otherwise specified as 2-surgeon.

Etiology

The most common cause of unilateral ankle arthritis is posttraumatic arthritis reported in 70% to 78% of cases.[1–3] This is dissimilar to knee and hip arthritis, which is most commonly due to osteoarthritis. Valderrabano and colleagues studied the causes of ankle arthritis in 390 patients and reported posttraumatic ankle arthritis represented 78% of the cases (n = 318), secondary arthritis 13% (n = 52), and primary osteoarthritis 9% (n = 36).[3] Similarly, Saltzman and colleagues reported that in a consecutive series of 639 patients with ankle arthritis, 70% (n = 445) were posttraumatic, 12% (n = 76) were secondary arthritis (rheumatoid disease), and 7% (n = 46) were primary osteoarthritis.[2] However, in the setting of bilateral ankle pathologic condition, there is a much higher rate of primary and secondary arthritis. Previous literature studying patients with bilateral ankle arthritis report the causes of up to 56% primary osteoarthritis[4] and 65% secondary arthritis.[1,5] The mental and physical disability associated with end-stage ankle arthritis is comparable to the morbidity of end-stage arthritis of the hip.[6] Additionally, bilateral ankle arthritis is a more debilitating condition with worse American Orthopedic Foot and Ankle Society (AOFAS) hindfoot and short-form 36 (SF-36) scores than unilateral disease.[1,5]

DISCUSSION
Bilateral Total Ankle Arthroplasty Literature

There are only 5 reports in the literature studying bilateral TAA that are outlined in **Table 1**.[1,4,5,7,8] Karantana and colleagues described the first case series of 5 patients who underwent bilateral Scandinavian Total Ankle Replacement (STAR) TAA (DJO Global, Lewisville, TX), performed in one operative setting by a single surgeon.[8] The authors reported 2 cases of delayed wound healing with superficial infection and one nondisplaced medial malleolus fracture, all which healed without return to the

Table 1
Bilateral total ankle arthroplasty literature

Author, Year	Surgery Dates	Follow-up, Mean	Prostheses	Setting	N patients	Postoperative protocol[a]	Outcomes at Final Follow-up[a]	Complications, per Ankle[a]
Karantana et al,[8] 2010	2002–2006	46 mo	STAR	1 Stage 1 Surgeon	5	Day 0–4: NWB, plaster splint; Day 4–Week 2: WBAT, plaster walking splint; Week 2–6: WBAT, Below-knee walking cast	AOFAS: 86; Satisfaction 100%; Total ROM: 8°; Hospital Stay: 4 d minimum	• 2 delayed wound healing; • 1 medial malleolus fracture; Reoperation: 0; Metal revision: 0
Barg et al,[5] 2010[b]	2001–2008	46 mo	HINTEGRA	1 Stage 1 Surgeon Unilateral TAA	23 46	Day 0–2: NWB, plaster splint; Day 2–Day 3 or 4: WBAT, below-knee walking cast; Day 3 or 4–Week 6: WBAT, stable walker	VAS: 1.7; AOFAS: 72; SF-36 PCS: 69.8; SF-36 MCS: 76.6; Total ROM: 39°; Hospital Stay: 7 d average	No complications reported; Reoperation: 0; Metal revision: 0
Barg et al,[7] 2011[b]	2000–2008	5.2 y	HINTEGRA	1 Stage 1 Surgeon	26	Same as above	VAS: 2.0; AOFAS: 74; SF-36 PCS: 68; SF-36 MCS: 73; ROM: 39°; Satisfaction: 100% (7 very satisfied, 16 satisfied, 3 satisfied with reservation)	• 1 delayed wound healing; • 4 component revisions for aseptic loosening; • 2 medial impingement pain; • 1 hindfoot valgus; Reoperation: 11.5%; Metal revision: 7.7%; Survival to component revision: 91% at 5 y; 78% at 8 y

(continued on next page)

Table 1
(continued)

Author, Year	Surgery Dates	Follow-up, Mean	Prostheses	Setting	N patients	Postoperative protocol[a]	Outcomes at Final Follow-up[a]	Complications, per Ankle[a]
Desai et al,[1] 2017	2002–2014	5.0 y	STAR Mobility HINTEGRA Agility	2 Stage (Average 486 d apart) Unilateral TAA	53 (37 included in the analysis) 106	Not specified	SF-36 PCS: 39.5 SF-36 MCS: 56 AAOS-FAM FAC: 80 AAOS-FAM SHOE: 58	• 6 removal or revision of metal components • 2 polyethylene liner exchange • 9 ancillary procedures Reoperation: 23% Metal revision: 8%
Fletcher et al,[4] 2022	2007–2019	52.2 mo	Vantage INBONE Salto Talaris STAR Infinity	1 Stage 2 Surgeon 2 Stage (Average 17.5 mo apart)	25 25	Week 0–3: WBAT, short leg walking cast Week 3–6: WBAT, CAM boot	1 Stage: VAS: 13.5 SF-36: 73.5 SMFA-F: 15.3 SMFA-B: 21.1 2 Stage: VAS:10.2 SF-36: 67.8 SMFA-F: 17.3 SMFA-B: 21.4	1 Stage: Complications: 22.0% Reoperations: 12% Metal revision: 2% (1 ankle at 8 y postoperative) 2 Stage: Complications: 24.0% Reoperations: 10% Metal revision: 0 5-y reoperation-free survival: 88.0% 1 Stage 90.0% 2 Stage 5-y failure-free survival: 100% both cohorts

Abbreviations: AAOS-FAM, American Academy of Orthopedic Surgeons Foot And Ankle Module; AOFAS, American Orthopedic Foot and Ankle Surgeons; CAM, controlled ankle motion; FAC, foot and ankle core scale; MCS, mental component summary; NWB, non–weight-bearing; PCS, physical component summary; ROM, range of motion; SF-36, short form 36; SHOE, shoe comfort scale; SMFA-B, short musculoskeletal function assessment bother index; SMFA-F, short musculoskeletal function assessment function index; STAR, Scandinavian total ankle replacement; VAS, visual analog scale; WBAT, weight-bearing as tolerated.

[a] Postoperative protocol, outcomes, and complications reported for bilateral TAA patients only.

[b] Same patient cohort, longer follow-up.

operating room. They reported a 100% satisfaction rate and mean postoperative AOFAS score of 86.

Barg and colleagues published both short-term[5] and later midterm[7] follow-ups on patients who underwent bilateral TAA in one operative setting by a single surgeon. At a minimum of 2 years follow-up, they included 23 patients who underwent simultaneous bilateral TAA in comparison to 46 matched patients who underwent unilateral TAA with the HINTEGRA prosthesis (Integra Life Sciences, Newdeal SA, Lyon, France). The authors concluded greater improvements in postoperative pain scores and patient-reported outcome measures (PROMs) in unilateral TAA patients in the immediate postoperative period; however, the outcomes were equivalent at 1-year and 2-year follow-ups compared with bilateral TAA. Barg and colleagues subsequently reported midterm follow-up on this bilateral cohort, including 26 patients or 52 ankles, at a minimum of 5 years postoperative.[7] The authors reported secondary reoperations in 6 ankles (11.5%), which included 4 (7.7%) prosthetic component revisions for aseptic loosening. With revision of any component for any reason as the endpoint, the survival rate was 91% at 5 years and 78% at 8 years.

Desai and colleagues studied the quality of life in 53 patients who underwent 2-stage bilateral TAA compared with 106 patients who underwent unilateral TAA at an average of 5 years follow-up. There was an average of 486 days between the first and second TAA in the bilateral patients. Despite a worse preoperative health status in the bilateral group, the 2 cohorts had equivalent improvement in PROMs, reoperations, and component survival rates. Thus, the authors concluded that patients who underwent staged bilateral TAA benefited as much as patients who underwent unilateral TAA, despite having a worse preoperative health status.

Most recently, the current author and colleagues evaluated the safety and efficacy of bilateral TAA comparing patients who underwent bilateral "simultaneous" (single-stage, 2-surgeon) versus "sequential" (2-stage) TAA including perioperative complications and PROMs at an average of 52 months follow-up. This was the first comparative study of single-stage versus 2-stage bilateral TAA in the ankle arthroplasty literature. This study was also unique in the fact that all bilateral surgeries were performed by 2 surgeon teams operating simultaneously, or in parallel, under one anesthetic event. In the aforementioned bilateral TAA studies, the bilateral surgeries were performed by one senior surgeon who performed the TAA sequentially, or one ankle at a time under the same anesthetic event. The authors confirmed prior studies that patients with bilateral ankle arthritis represent a unique population with a higher incidence of primary osteoarthritis compared with earlier reports of patients with unilateral pathologic condition. All patients undergoing bilateral TAA showed significant improvements in pain and PROMs postoperatively. When comparing single-stage 2-surgeon versus 2-stage bilateral TAA, there were no significant differences in PROMs, pain, or perioperative complication rates. There were similar total complications (22.0% vs 24.0%), intraoperative complications (2.0% medial malleolus fracture vs 2.0% burn with electrocautery), reoperations (6.0% vs 5.0%), component revisions (2.0% vs 0%), reoperation-free survival, and failure-free survival between the single-stage 2-surgeon and 2-stage cohorts, respectively. Overall, the authors advocated that simultaneous bilateral TAA is a safe and effective method for the treatment of bilateral end-stage ankle arthritis. Figs. 1 and 2 provide radiographic examples of bilateral TAA performed via the 2-stage and single-stage 1-surgeon techniques, respectively.

Indications

There are no well-established indications or contraindications for consideration of simultaneous bilateral TAA. Patient selection is multifactorial and often a subjective

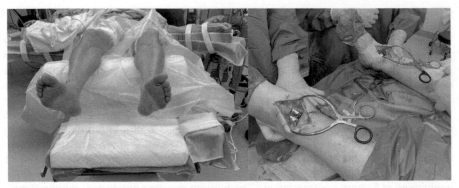

Fig. 1. Patient positioning for single-stage, 2-surgeon bilateral TAAs. The patient is positioned with the feet at the end of the table, and an arm board is placed parallel at the distal end of the table to increase the operating space.

decision made by both the patient and surgeon. Considerations including timing of symptom onset and progression, comorbidities, patient preference, patient endurance, home support, and surgeon and staff expertise must be evaluated during operative planning. Given the different risk–benefit profiles of single-stage versus 2-stage procedures, potential complications must be interpreted in light of each individual patient. Typically, simultaneous surgery is considered in patients who are younger, have adequate bone quality, few comorbidities, are self-motivated, have the endurance to mobilize with bilateral postoperative immobilization, and have appropriate social support at home to ensure safety during the recovery period. Following simultaneous surgery, patients are typically permitted to immediately weight-bear as tolerated in short leg casts. Thus, patients must not require concomitant procedures that would necessitate non–weight-bearing postoperatively. One recommendation is to offer

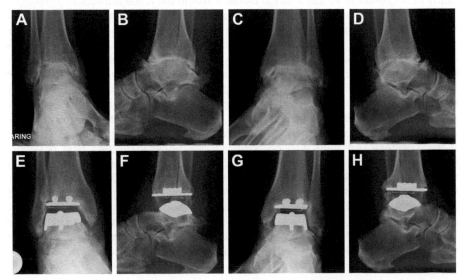

Fig. 2. Preoperative anterior-posterior (*A, C*) and lateral (*B, D*) radiographs and 7-year postoperative anterior-posterior (*E, G*) and lateral (*F, H*) radiographs of a 67-year-old man who underwent staged TAA with STAR (DJO Global, Lewisville, TX) prostheses. The right and left TAAs were performed 1 year apart.

preoperative physical therapy to practice safe mobility with bilateral lower extremity immobilization using controlled ankle motion (CAM) boots.

In a systematic review of simultaneous bilateral versus staged total hip arthroplasty (THA), the authors concluded that the available evidence supports the performance of simultaneous bilateral THA in selected patients (aged <65 years, American Society of Anesthesiology score 1–2, without cardiovascular comorbidities) and suggests the avoidance of staged surgeries within the same hospitalization.[9] Although no sound evidence, these may be important considerations for ankle arthroplasty as well. Patients undergoing staged arthroplasty are typically counseled preoperatively that the contralateral TAA may be performed as early as 3 to 6 months postoperatively pending their recovery.

Operative Technique and Postoperative Protocol

When discussing bilateral TAA, this may be performed in a single-stage (1 operative event) or 2-stage fashion (2 operative events). The single-stage surgery may be performed by a single surgeon team performing the procedures one after the other in the same operative setting or by 2 surgical teams operating in parallel. There is only one previous study reporting single-stage 2-surgeon bilateral TAA with surgeries performed under one anesthetic event.[4] In the other bilateral TAA studies, the surgeries were performed in a single-stage 1-surgeon manner with one senior surgeon and operative team performing the TAA one ankle at a time under a single anesthetic event.[1,5,7]

The surgical technique for single-stage 2-surgeon bilateral TAA has been previously described.[4] Regional anesthesia with bilateral popliteal and adductor canal nerve blocks are administered by the anesthesia team. To increase the operating space, a radiolucent arm board is placed parallel at the distal end of the operative table (**Fig. 3**). One or 2 arm boards on each side of the table may be placed. The patient is then positioned supine with their feet at the end of the table. This setup allows both surgical teams to operate from the table end. Bilateral thigh tourniquets are placed and are inflated simultaneously at the

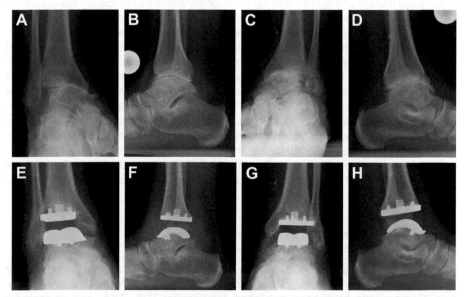

Fig. 3. Preoperative anterior-posterior (A, C) and lateral (B, D) radiographs and 5-year postoperative anterior-posterior (E, G) and lateral (F, H) radiographs of a 78-year-old man who underwent bilateral 1-stage 2-surgeon TAA with Vantage (Exactech, Gainesville, FL) prostheses.

start of the procedure. However, it is recommended that the tourniquets are sequentially deflated with a minimum of 5 minutes between deflation to prevent a rapid shift in intravascular volume. A single C-arm x-ray machine is used during the surgery, positioned at either side of the operating table where it will remain for the duration of the case. A radiology technician will control the C-arm for the surgeons. The TAAs are then performed based on standard technique and the manufacturers' technique protocol. Concomitant surgeries are performed as needed to achieve appropriate component alignment, ankle stability, and foot alignment. To reemphasize, no surgeries that necessitate non–weight-bearing postoperatively should be performed, requiring thoughtful preoperative planning.

In terms of the postoperative protocol, both immediate weight-bearing[4] and a few days of non–weight-bearing followed by weight-bearing as tolerated[1,5,7,8] have been described. In the initial reports of bilateral TAA, the patients maintained non–weight-bearing in a splint or cast for 3 to 4 days postoperative, which were then changed to plaster walking casts[8] or a stable walker[5,7] with permissible weight-bearing as tolerated. More recently, the postoperative protocol recommended is immediate immobilization in short-leg walking casts for 3 weeks.[4] The patients are allowed to immediately weight-bear as tolerated. Patients return to clinic at 3 weeks postoperatively for wound inspection and suture removal. At that time, they transition into removable below-the-knee CAM boots, which they use for an additional 3 weeks. During this time, patients initiate self-directed ankle motion exercises. At 6 weeks postoperative, patients wean out of the CAM boots and begin weight-bearing as tolerated in normal shoe wear. Patients return for postoperative follow-up at 3 weeks, 6 weeks, 3 months, 6 months, 1 year, and annually thereafter. To date, no literature has evaluated or compared postoperative protocols following TAA. However, there are anecdotal reports of immediate partial or full weight-bearing following either bilateral or unilateral TAA without observed increased complications.[4,10]

Although there is ample knee and hip arthroplasty literature comparing the outcomes between single-stage versus 2-stage bilateral arthroplasty, there is only one study comparing the single-stage 1-surgeon (1 surgeon sequential) versus single-stage 2-surgeon (2 surgeons simultaneous) techniques.[11] In this recent prospective randomized controlled trial of bilateral total knee arthroplasty (TKA), Uzer and colleagues demonstrated no difference in short-term radiologic and functional outcomes between the 2 cohorts. In fact, the authors reported a lower major complication rate and operative times in the 2-surgeon TKA group. Thus, they concluded that single-stage 2-surgeon simultaneous bilateral TKA is as safe as single-stage 1-surgeon sequential bilateral TKA. Additionally, Qadir and colleagues indicated that there were no significant differences in component alignment between the first or second knee in single-stage 1-surgeon sequential bilateral TKA and unilateral TKA.[12] There have been no previous reports comparing radiographic outcomes of bilateral 2-stage, single-stage 1-surgeon simultaneous, single-stage 1-surgeon sequential, or unilateral TAAs.

HIP AND KNEE ARTHROPLASTY LITERATURE
Risks and Benefits of Bilateral Arthroplasty

Aside from the aforementioned 5 studies on bilateral ankle arthroplasty, much of our current knowledge on bilateral joint arthroplasty comes from the hip and knee literature. Comparisons have been published for bilateral THA, TKA, and unicondylar knee arthroplasty (UKA). These include case series of bilateral arthroplasty, comparison of bilateral to unilateral arthroplasty, and direct comparisons of bilateral simultaneous versus 2-stage arthroplasty. Those in support of simultaneous bilateral arthroplasty note significant cost savings, noninferior and even superior perioperative complication profiles, improved PROM and satisfaction, shorter total recovery time, early rehabilitation, and less time away from employment when compared with unilateral or staged procedures.

Two large systematic reviews and meta-analyses were conducted to compare simultaneous versus 2-stage bilateral TKA, both including 18 studies.[13,14] These studies report benefits of simultaneous bilateral TKA including a lower risk of deep infection and respiratory complications. Liu and colleagues also found lower revision rates in the simultaneous group, whereas Fu and colleagues found no difference. However, these benefits are at the risk of an increased 30-day mortality, pulmonary embolism (PE), and blood transfusion rates compared with bilateral staged TKA. Liu and colleagues also found a higher rate of deep venous thrombosis (DVT) in the simultaneous group, whereas Fu and colleagues found no difference. Both studies found no significant differences in superficial infection, arthrofibrosis, cardiac complications, neurologic complications, and urinary complications between procedures. The theoretic benefits of simultaneous bilateral arthroplasty performed under a single anesthetic event are numerous and extend beyond the perioperative complication profile. In a systematic review of 10 studies reporting functional outcomes following simultaneous versus staged bilateral TKA, Qadir and colleagues reported moderate evidence to suggest equivalent improvement in functional outcome scores in the simultaneous bilateral cohort.[12] Additionally, another systematic review including 8 studies of patients undergoing simultaneous bilateral UKA reported reduction in the operating time, length of stay, and hospital cost without increasing postoperative complications compared with staged bilateral UKA.[15]

Somewhat dissimilar to the above are 2 a systematic reviews and meta-analyses conducted for simultaneous versus staged bilateral THA.[16,17] In a the review including 38 studies, Ramezani and colleagues reported a significant reduction in DVT, total blood loss, and systemic, local, and pulmonary complications in the simultaneous bilateral group.[17] However, there was an increased PE and periprosthetic fracture risk. The authors also reported a reduction in the total length of hospital stay and total cost in the simultaneous bilateral group. Huang and colleagues included 19 studies in their review and found the simultaneous bilateral THA was associated with a reduction in the occurrence of DVT, PE, and respiratory complications.[16] However, there was no significant difference between the groups in terms of mortality. As highlighted in the above findings, although there is ample bilateral hip and knee arthroplasty literature, the findings are largely inconsistent with multiple individual studies and even the meta-analyses reporting conflicting risk–benefit profiles of each approach. This further challenges the ability to infer any trends onto bilateral ankle arthroplasty.

When extrapolating the above findings of knee and hip arthroplasty, particularly the increased risk of thromboembolic events and blood transfusions in simultaneous bilateral arthroplasty, it is important to consider the differences of ankle arthroplasty. Although increased blood loss and transfusion rates may be seen with knee and hip arthroplasty, ankle arthroplasty is almost exclusively performed with a tourniquet. Regional anesthesia has also been shown to reduce both blood loss and the incidence of DVT compared with general anesthesia in elective hip and knee surgery.[18,19] Additionally, many of the studies were performed before routine tranexamic acid use. Tranexamic acid use is associated with lower estimated blood loss in foot and ankle surgeries without an increased risk of thromboembolic events, wound complications, or changes in hemoglobin.[20] Thus, the use of regional anesthesia, tourniquets, and tranexamic acid may help mitigate the risk of thromboembolic events and blood transfusions in bilateral TAA seen in the bilateral hip and knee literature.

Cost of Bilateral Arthroplasty

One of the distinguishing factors of the simultaneous bilateral arthroplasty procedure is overall cost reduction and anesthesia time. An older study from 1998 evaluating the inpatient cost comparison of simultaneous bilateral arthroplasty to unilateral arthroplasty reported a 25% reduction in cost which translates to ~US$10,000 for each TKA patient and more than US$8000 for each THA patient.[21] However, cost considerations must include total cost (cost to the patient and health-care system as a whole when including inpatient and outpatient care) rather than hospitalization cost alone. More recently published, Odum and colleagues reported the estimated average cost in 2012 US dollar to be US$43,401 for a simultaneous bilateral TKA compared with US$72,233 for staged bilateral TKA.[22] Their analysis included hospital cost, rehabilitation costs, anesthesia costs, physician fees, and heath utilities. The largest percent (55%) of total cost savings from a hospital perspective has been attributed to the cost of operating room staff and setup.[23] No similar cost comparison studies have been performed for bilateral ankle arthroplasty. However, when considering the financial burden on society, patient selection and complication probability must be thoughtfully reviewed when considering bilateral arthroplasty procedures.

Single-Stage 1-Surgeon Versus 2-Surgeon Technique

The single-stage 1-surgeon versus 2-surgeon team bilateral arthroplasty techniques have been compared in the TKA literature. In a recent prospective randomized controlled trial by Uzer and colleagues, the authors demonstrated no difference in short-term radiologic and functional outcomes between the 2 cohorts undergoing bilateral TKA.[11] Although the 2-surgeon team had greater estimated blood loss, there was also shorter operative times and a lower 90-day major complication rate than the 1-surgeon bilateral TKA group. The authors concluded that single-stage 2-surgeon bilateral TKA is safe with lower complication rates than single-stage 1-surgeon bilateral TKA. Similarly, in the study by Fletcher and colleagues comparing single-stage 2-surgeon bilateral TAA to 2-stage TAA, there were no increased intraoperative or total complications with similar PROMs and survivability.[4]

SUMMARY

Patients with bilateral ankle arthritis are more likely to have primary osteoarthritis or secondary inflammatory arthritis than patients with unilateral ankle arthritis. Additionally, patients with bilateral ankle arthritis have a more debilitation condition with worse PROMs and health-related quality of life (HRQOL) than patients with unilateral ankle arthritis. Considerations for indicating a patient for bilateral TAA include the patient's age, bone health, comorbidities, concomitant procedures required (should not necessitate non–weight-bearing postoperative), home support, self-motivation, endurance to mobilize with bilateral postoperative immobilization, and surgeon and team experience. Perioperative considerations for bilateral TAA include regional anesthesia, thigh tourniquets with sequential deflation at least 5 minutes apart, tranexamic acid, parallel arm board(s) at the end of the table to increase the operating space, and immediate postoperative weight-bearing as tolerated in short leg casts, which has not been show to result in increased complication rates. There is limited literature evaluating bilateral TAA with studies limited to small retrospective analyses. However, in general, the literature supports both 1-surgeon and 2-surgeon team bilateral TAA as safe and effective with comparable improvements in PROMs, complications, reoperations, and prosthesis survival as unilateral TAA and 2-stage bilateral TAA. The more robust bilateral knee and hip arthroplasty literature further highlights potential risks (increased intraoperative blood loss and thromboembolic events) and benefits (cost reduction, noninferior and even superior perioperative complication profiles, improved PROMs and satisfaction, shorter total recovery time, early rehabilitation, and less time away from employment) of bilateral arthroplasty when compared with unilateral or staged procedures. In conclusion, when performed under surgeon expertise in appropriately selected patients, simultaneous bilateral TAA is a safe and effective method for the treatment of bilateral end-stage ankle arthritis. However, larger studies should expand on the potential risks and benefits, specifically evaluating radiographic outcomes, further clinical outcomes, perioperative complications, surgery time, tourniquet time, length of hospitalization, recovery and rehabilitation time, days of work missed, overall cost, and others.

CLINICS CARE POINTS

- Patients with bilateral ankle arthritis have higher rates of primary and secondary/ inflammatory arthritis and a more debilitating condition (worse PROMs and health-related quality of life) than those with unilateral pathologic condition.

- Considerations for indicating a patient for bilateral TAA include the patient's age, bone health, comorbidities, concomitant procedures required (should not necessitate non–weight-bearing postoperative), home support, self-motivation, endurance to mobilize with bilateral postoperative immobilization, and surgeon and team experience.

- Perioperative considerations for bilateral TAA include regional anesthesia, thigh tourniquets with sequential deflation at least 5 minutes apart, tranexamic acid, parallel arm board at the end of the table to increase the operating space, and immediate postoperative weight-bearing as tolerated in short leg casts, which has not been show to result in increased complication rates.

- The limited bilateral TAA literature supports both 1-surgeon and 2-surgeon team bilateral TAAs as safe and effective with comparable improvements in PROMs, complications, reoperations, and prosthesis survival as unilateral TAA and 2-stage bilateral TAA.

- The more robust bilateral knee and hip arthroplasty literature further highlights potential risks (increased intraoperative blood loss and thromboembolic events) and benefits (cost reduction, noninferior and even superior perioperative complication profiles, improved PROMs and satisfaction, shorter total recovery time, early rehabilitation, and less time away from employment) of bilateral arthroplasty when compared with unilateral or staged procedures.

ACKNOWLEDGMENT

The author thanks Dr James DeOrio, Dr James (Jim) Nunley, and Dr Mark Easley for allowing the study of their patients and use of patient images and radiographs.

DISCLOSURES

The author has nothing to disclose.

REFERENCES

1. Desai SJ, Glazebrook M, Penner MJ, et al. Quality of Life in Bilateral Vs. Unilateral End-Stage Ankle Arthritis and Outcomes of Bilateral Vs. Unilateral Total Ankle Replacement. J Bone Joint Surg Am 2017;99(2):133–40.

2. Saltzman CL, Salamon ML, Blanchard GM, et al. Epidemiology of ankle arthritis: report of a consecutive series of 639 patients from a tertiary orthopaedic center. Iowa Orthop J 2005;25:44–6.
3. Valderrabano V, Horisberger M, Russell I, et al. Etiology of ankle osteoarthritis. Clin Orthop Relat Res 2009;467(7):1800–6.
4. Fletcher AN, Johnson LG, Easley ME, et al. Clinical Outcomes and Complications of Simultaneous or Sequential Bilateral Total Ankle Arthroplasty: A Single-Center Comparative Cohort Study. J Bone Joint Surg Am 2022;104(19):1712–21.
5. Barg A, Knupp M, Hintermann B. Simultaneous bilateral versus unilateral total ankle replacement: a patient-based comparison of pain relief, quality of life and functional outcome. J Bone Joint Surg Br 2010;92(12):1659–63.
6. Glazebrook M, Daniels T, Younger A, et al. Comparison of health-related quality of life between patients with end-stage ankle and hip arthrosis. J Bone Joint Surg Am 2008;90(3):499–505.
7. Barg A, Henninger HB, Knupp M, et al. Simultaneous bilateral total ankle replacement using a 3-component prosthesis: outcome in 26 patients followed for 2–10 years. Acta Orthop 2011;82(6):704–10.
8. Karantana A, Martin Geoghegan J, Shandil M, et al. Simultaneous bilateral total ankle replacement using the S.T.A.R.: a case series. Foot Ankle Int 2010; 31(1):86–9.
9. Muskus M, Rojas J, Gutiérrez C, et al. Bilateral Hip Arthroplasty: When Is It Safe to Operate the Second Hip? A Systematic Review. BioMed Res Int 2018;2018: 3150349.
10. Usuelli FG, Paoli T, Indino C, et al. Fast-Track for Total Ankle Replacement: A Novel Enhanced Recovery Protocol for Select Patients. Foot Ankle Int 2023; 44(2):148–58.
11. Uzer G, Aliyev O, Yıldız F, et al. Safety of one-stage bilateral total knee arthroplasty -one surgeon sequential vs. two surgeons simultaneous: a randomized controlled study. Int Orthop 2020;44(10):2009–15.
12. Qadir I, Shah B, Waqas M, et al. Component Alignment in Simultaneous Bilateral versus Unilateral Total Knee Arthroplasty. Knee Surg Relat Res 2019;31(1):31–6.
13. Fu D, Li G, Chen K, et al. Comparison of clinical outcome between simultaneous-bilateral and staged-bilateral total knee arthroplasty: a systematic review of retrospective studies. J Arthroplasty 2013;28(7):1141–7.
14. Liu L, Liu H, Zhang H, et al. Bilateral total knee arthroplasty: Simultaneous or staged? A systematic review and meta-analysis. Medicine (Baltim) 2019; 98(22):e15931.
15. Chen W, Sun J, Zhang Y, et al. Staged vs simultaneous bilateral unicompartmental knee arthroplasty for clinical outcomes: A protocol of systematic review and meta-analysis. Medicine (Baltim) 2021;100(14):e25240.
16. Huang L, Xu T, Li P, et al. Comparson of mortality and complications between bilateral simultaneous and staged total hip arthroplasty: A systematic review and meta-analysis. Medicine (Baltim) 2019;98(39):e16774.
17. Ramezani A, Ghaseminejad Raeini A, Sharafi A, et al. Simultaneous versus staged bilateral total hip arthroplasty: a systematic review and meta-analysis. J Orthop Surg Res 2022;17(1):392.
18. Davis FM, Laurenson VG, Gillespie WJ, et al. Deep vein thrombosis after total hip replacement. A comparison between spinal and general anaesthesia. J Bone Joint Surg Br 1989;71(2):181–5.

19. Sharrock NE, Haas SB, Hargett MJ, et al. Effects of epidural anesthesia on the incidence of deep-vein thrombosis after total knee arthroplasty. J Bone Joint Surg Am 1991;73(4):502–6.
20. Salameh M, Attia AK, El Khatib S, et al. Tranexamic Acid Utilization in Foot and Ankle Surgery: A Meta-analysis. Foot Ankle Int 2022;43(10):1370–8.
21. Reuben JD, Meyers SJ, Cox DD, et al. Cost comparison between bilateral simultaneous, staged, and unilateral total joint arthroplasty. J Arthroplasty 1998;13(2):172–9.
22. Odum SM, Troyer JL, Kelly MP, et al. A cost-utility analysis comparing the cost-effectiveness of simultaneous and staged bilateral total knee arthroplasty. J Bone Joint Surg Am 2013;95(16):1441–9.
23. Martin GR, Marsh JD, Vasarhelyi EM, et al. A cost analysis of single-stage bilateral versus two-stage direct anterior total hip arthroplasty. Hip Int 2016; 26(1):15–9.

Outcomes of Total Ankle Arthroplasty After Reoperation due to Gutter Impingement

Jaeyoung Kim, MD[1], Constantine Demetracopoulos, MD*

KEYWORDS

- Total ankle arthroplasty • Ankle arthritis • Gutter impingement • Reoperation
- Weight-bearing computed tomography • Complication

KEY POINTS

- Gutter impingement is one of the most common causes that leads to subsequent surgery after total ankle arthroplasty (TAA).
- Most literature indicates the resolution of gutter impingement symptoms after gutter debridement. However, its longer term efficacy is questionable because residual pain, recurrence of symptoms, and poorer functional outcome scores have been described in gutter debridement patients.
- Gutter impingement may be due to inadequate debridement at the time of TAA. However, it may also be a manifestation of TAA malalignment or residual deformity in the foot. Therefore, a thorough physical examination and the use of advanced imaging modalities are required to optimize initial component alignment and foot realignment, as well as subsequent procedures for managing gutter impingement symptoms.

INTRODUCTION

The number of total ankle arthroplasty (TAA) being performed in the United States is increasing with the advent of new implants, and an improved understanding of the biomechanics of the foot and ankle and the surgical techniques are necessary for successful TAA.[1–3] Although the revision rate, indicating implant failure, has decreased during the years, the rate of subsequent surgery due to nonrevisional causes following index TAA remains significant.[4–12] According to a recent systematic review, the need for subsequent surgery was the most notable difference between TAA and ankle arthrodesis.[13] This suggests that reducing the incidence of subsequent surgery is

---

Foot and Ankle Service, Hospital for Special Surgery, New York, NY, USA
[1] Present address: 532 east 72nd Street, New York, NY.
* Corresponding author. 535 East 70th Street, New York, NY 10021.
E-mail address: demetracopoulosc@hss.edu

Foot Ankle Clin N Am 29 (2024) 111–122
https://doi.org/10.1016/j.fcl.2023.08.005
1083-7515/24/© 2023 Elsevier Inc. All rights reserved.

important in making TAA a more reliable treatment option for both surgeons and patients with end-stage ankle arthritis. A comprehensive understanding of the causes of subsequent surgeries after TAA and their prevention is still needed.

Gutter impingement is widely considered the most common cause of subsequent surgery after TAA, with incidence rates ranging from 6% to 45%.[14–18] It was also found to be the most common cause of complications after TAA in a recent meta-analysis, with a pooled rate of 0.06 (95% CI 0.04–0.08).[19] Although both open and arthroscopic debridement can provide short-term relief of symptoms,[20–22] recurrence has been reported after surgical intervention.[21,22] A recent study also found that patient-reported outcomes at midterm follow-up were worse for those who underwent impingement-associated reoperation compared with those who did not.[20] The aforementioned findings raise the question whether our current approach adequately addresses the root causes of gutter impingement. This article discusses the causes of gutter impingement, the indications for surgical treatment, and the results of reoperation due to gutter impingement following TAA.

CAUSES OF GUTTER IMPINGEMENT

Gutter impingement is a condition that can cause persistent pain in the ankle after TAA. It occurs when the talar implant, or the native talar bone, impinges against the medial or lateral malleolus. The causes of gutter impingement can be complex and interrelated and can include factors such as the design and characteristics of the implant, its alignment and position, and the formation of heterotopic bone.[23] Soft tissue impingement can also be a factor.[24] As is well known, the cause of gutter impingement is multifactorial; therefore, a thorough physical examination and correlation with radiographic or advanced imaging findings, such as weight-bearing computed tomography (WBCT) or single-photon-emission computed tomography (SPECT)-CT,[25] can help identify potential causes of gutter impingement.

Implant Characteristics

The difference in the design rationale of the implant in each system can contribute to the development of impingement. Each implant system has a unique understanding of the morphologic characteristics of the articulating surfaces of the ankle joint,[26] and the resultant ankle kinematics following implantation can contribute to the development of gutter impingement. It is also important to consider the altered kinematics of bones due to changes in gait patterns or abnormal rotation of the talus in ankle arthritis,[27–29] which can possibly be addressed through implantation technique itself or concurrent procedures at the time of TAA.

The design of the implant apparently influences the development of gutter impingement, as demonstrated by the Agility TAA system.[30] The Agility system replaces both the medial and lateral malleoli and has a narrower talus compared with the tibial component and has been shown to have a lower incidence of gutter impingement in the early postoperative period. However, as reported by Shuberth and colleagues,[22] impingement can occur at a relatively later interval after implantation compared with other systems, when subsidence of the talar component causes the undersides of the tibial component to encroach on the native talar bone. Additionally, this system has shown higher rates (45% of 127 reoperations) of heterotopic ossification formation, requiring debridement at a mean follow-up of 33 months for 306 patients, as reported by Spirt and colleagues[7]

The limited number of comparative studies makes it difficult to determine the exact incidence of gutter disease among various ankle implants. Rajan and colleagues compared the midterm outcomes of 44 INBONE II (Wright Medical Group, Memphis, TN) and 85 Salto Talaris (Integra, Plainsboro, NJ) TAA patients and found that the Salto Talaris patients had a higher reoperation rate, largely due to gutter impingement (66.6% of all reoperation causes).[11] They speculated that the difference may have been due to the design of the talar component, with the Salto Talaris talus having a conical shape with 2 different radii of curvature and INBONE II having a symmetric bicondylar design. However, they acknowledged that the difference could not be solely attributed to the implant design because preoperative deformity and surgeon factors could also have influenced the reoperation rate.

The type of polyethylene insert used in TAA can potentially influence the development of gutter impingement. Mobile-bearing TAA was thought to have a higher likelihood of impingement due to the increased freedom of motion between the tibial component and insert, which allows for mediolateral subluxation.[30] However, recent studies have shown minimal movement of the insert in mobile-bearing implants,[31,32] making the earlier assumption uncertain. The literature is inconclusive on the difference between the 2 types of bearings, with a prospective randomized trial by Nunely and colleagues finding similar rates of gutter impingement between mobile-bearing STAR (Stryker, Kalamazoo, MI) and fixed-bearing Salto Talaris TAA systems.[33] Nevertheless, studies have shown medial translation of the talus after mobile-bearing TAA with malalignment of the varus tibial implant or valgus hindfoot,[34–36] suggesting that the mobile-bearing system may be susceptible to gutter impingement if the implant or foot alignment are not well balanced.

The relationship between the type of surgical approach and the occurrence of gutter impingement has also been explored. Oliver and colleagues found a higher rate of postoperative gutter impingement in patients who underwent TAA using the lateral approach Trabecular Metal TAA system (Zimmer Biomet, Warsaw, Indiana) compared with those who underwent TAA using the anterior approach (INFINITY [Wright Medical Group, Memphis, TN] and INBONE).[37] This difference may be due to the limited ability to debride the medial gutter during the lateral approach, leading to insufficient space between the implant and the medial malleolus. To overcome this, surgeons who use a lateral approach implant will often make a separate anteromedial incision to adequately debride the medial gutter. Further research in this area may provide a better understanding of the relationship between surgical approach and gutter impingement.

Besides the inherent design of the implant, the size of the implant should be correctly chosen during surgery to avoid gutter impingement. Overstuffing the ankle mortise with a talar component that is too wide can cause impingement and restrict range of motion.[23] An oversized tibial implant may cause lateral impingement symptom due to impingement of the fibula at the syndesmosis or soft tissue impingement posteromedially against the posterior tibial tendon. Although a smaller talar component may reduce the risk of gutter encroachment, it may also cause impingement if subsidence occurs from excessive load on a relatively small talar component.[38] The thickness of the polyethylene insert also plays a crucial role because it affects the coronal height of the joint line and the talomalleolar distance. A thinner insert can result in hypermobility and mechanical impingement, as well as soft tissue impingement from hypertrophic scar tissue or synovium. Increasing the thickness can distract the gutters but may also lead to a reduced range of motion of the ankle, so careful evaluation during the surgery is necessary to find the optimal-sized polyethylene insert.

Inadequate Gutter Resection

Most implant systems do not include routine resection of both gutters in their manual. However, a study by Shuberth and colleagues showed that prophylactic resection of the gutter can decrease the incidence of gutter impingement.[22] In their study, 2% of patients who underwent prophylactic gutter resection during their index TAA experienced gutter impingement, compared with 7% of those who did not. The senior author of the study performs prophylactic gutter resection regardless of implant system when there is overhang at the talar side after implantation, using a reciprocating saw blade. It is advisable to visualize both the medial and lateral gutters with orthogonal views using intraoperative fluoroscopy to avoid impingement at the talomalleolar space. A portion of the medial malleolus or the medial aspect of the fibula may also be removed with a reciprocating saw to alleviate impingement. In contrast, Najefi and colleagues described the possible downsides of prophylactic gutter debridement such as concerns about instability of TAA within the ankle mortise, increased risk of malleolar fractures, and possible negative impact on future revision surgery from unnecessary bone resection.[39] They rather advocated that customizing the axial plane tibial component to patient-specific manner can decrease the rate of gutter impingement without preemptive resection.

Malalignment/Malrotation

Varus or valgus malalignment of the tibial component can increase the translation of the talus, leading to impingement symptoms due to their direct impact on talomalleolar distance or changes in kinematics (**Fig. 1**). Even if the components are properly aligned in the coronal plane, malalignment of the hindfoot or lower limb as a whole can affect the translation of the talus in the coronal plane, particularly in mobile-bearing systems, causing gutter impingement.[34–36] Devos Bevernage and colleagues described a patient with medial impingement after a mobile-bearing TAA and found that the patient had hindfoot valgus, which might have caused the talus to translate medially.[35] They performed a supramalleolar varus correction and hindfoot fusion, which eventually resolved the patient's symptoms. Yi and colleagues reported changes in the position of the talus after mobile-bearing TAA during a minimum 3-year period and found that postoperative talar translation in the coronal plane is correlated with preoperative talar translation, suggesting that concurrent realignment procedures for coronal plane malalignment may be necessary.[36] They also found that a varus lower limb mechanical axis, which affects the slope of the tibial plafond, and hindfoot valgus were associated with medial translation of the talus.

The mediolateral position of the component may also be a potential factor for gutter impingement. Saito and colleagues reported that the Salto Talaris fixed-bearing TAA system leads to greater internal rotation of the talus after implantation while reproducing normal ankle kinematics in the coronal and sagittal plane in a robotic gait cadaveric model.[40] They found that the medial-lateral position of the tibial component correlated with the amount of abnormal internal rotation of the talus during gait, which could play a significant role in medial gutter impingement.

Axial plane rotation is suggested to be one of the causes of postoperative impingement in TAA but it has not been widely investigated. With the advent of WBCT, the information regarding axial plane alignment of the distal tibia and talus, as well as the rotational profile of the implant, is now more accessible. Naefji and colleagues found a wide range of tibial torsion in ankle arthritis patients and a wide variance between 2 common axial rotation guide plans: the medial gutter line and the transmalleolar axis.[39] This suggests that current TAA referencing systems have the potential to lead to malpositioning of the tibial implant in the axial plane. They reported a lower incidence of gutter impingement after they started customizing axial plane alignment of the tibial component based on their preoperative CT scans. They described 3 out of 10 of their early cases that demonstrated medial impingement as having internal rotation of the

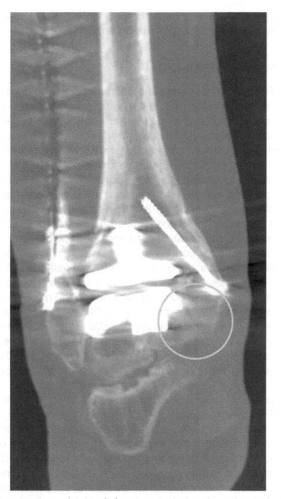

Fig. 1. A WBCT image was obtained from a patient who reported persistent medial impingement pain subsequent to Salto Talaris TAA. The image demonstrated a varus alignment of the tibial component, along with the presence of medial tibial and talar spurs that were causing impingement.

tibial component. More studies are needed regarding the axial plane alignment in TAA, from the rotational profile of the distal tibial plafond in patients with ankle arthritis to the ideal alignment of the tibial and talar implant in the TAA system in order to minimize postoperative impingement.

Soft Tissue Impingement

This refers to a condition where synovitis or scar tissue is entrapped between the joint space or opposing structures in the joint, causing pain. Hypertrophic scar tissue or synovitis can theoretically develop idiopathically or due to secondary causes, such as ligament imbalancing, loose bodies, or wear particles, leading to the development of secondary synovitis or hypertrophic scar tissue formation.[24,41] This can also be caused by the tendons around the joint. Krup and colleagues reported 2 cases of soft tissue impingement caused by the posterior tibial tendon, in which their decompression led to the resolution of the impingement symptoms.[14]

INDICATION OF SURGICAL TREATMENT

Ankle pain after TAA is not uncommon and characterizing it as impingement can often be challenging. Patients with impingement may complain of pain in the gutter area but pain from other sources such as sinus tarsi or subfibular impingement or posterior tibial tendon irritation should also be suspected. This is often accompanied by pain while walking and during palpation but gutter pain may be more likely to be associated with activity and relieved by rest.[22] Pain from gutter impingement can be very debilitating, and often needs to be distinguished from pain due to early loosening or subsidence. Although patients may report decreased range of motion, a study has shown that range of motion does not typically increase after gutter debridement.[42]

The efficacy of diagnostic injections is also unestablished. Injections can be used for therapeutic purposes to the suspected area of impingement. They can also be used to rule out extra-articular causes such as sinus tarsi impingement or tendon irritations. Pain relief following injection in the gutters of patients with impingement not only confirms the diagnosis but also indicates a good prognosis for debridement. However, injections should be used cautiously due to the risk of periprosthetic infection. It is our practice to wait at least 1 year after total ankle replacement before considering an injection for gutter impingement. We prefer an anesthetic only injection for diagnostic purposes but can consider one injection of corticosteroid for select patients in the hopes that the pain resolves. We do not recommend the use of repeated corticosteroid injections for gutter impingement due to the concern for prosthetic infection.

Plain radiographs may have limited value in visualizing impingement, unless it is clearly evident. Even when heterotopic ossification or spur impingement is present, it may not always be the source of the patient's symptoms. Unfortunately, a clear gutter finding on plain radiographs does not guarantee the absence of gutter impingement, as the static nature of these images may not reflect the dynamic nature of impingement that occurs during activities such as walking, running, or squatting. Advanced imaging techniques can provide additional support in making a diagnosis (Fig. 2). Mason and colleagues found a disparity between findings from SPECT-CT scans and plain radiographs in a study of 14 patients with painful TAA.[43] They discovered that although 13 cases showed prosthetic loosening/failure of bony ingrowth on SPECT-CT, only 10 of those cases showed evidence of loosening on plain radiographs. The potential benefits of using SPECT-CT were also described in a study that sought to correlate clinical and intraoperative findings in patients with painful TAA.[25] The authors of the study found a high degree of consistency between SPECT-CT results and clinical diagnosis, as well as intraoperative findings during revision surgery. Notably, they found that SPECT-CT yielded better consistency with clinical findings compared with MRI. WBCT, which provides a 3-dimensional analysis of the implant, foot-ankle alignment, and rotational profile of the implant in the axial plane, may be more helpful than conventional CT scans.

Once a diagnosis of gutter impingement has been made through imaging, it is important to assess other potential sources of pain and to evaluate the tibial and talar components for any signs of abnormality such as cyst formation, subsidence, loosening, changes in joint line height, or subluxation. This information will determine the type of subsequent surgery, whether it is a revision or nonrevisional reoperation, and whether an arthroscopic or open approach is required.

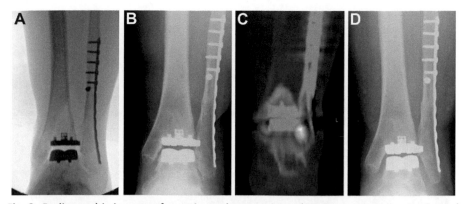

Fig. 2. Radiographic images of a patient who experienced gutter impingement pain and underwent gutter debridement after Vantage TAA. (*A*) Intraoperative fluoroscopic image immediately after TAA. (*B*) Weight-bearing ankle anteroposterior (AP) view 6 months post-TAA shows narrowed talomalleolar space on both the medial and lateral sides. (*C*) Single-photon emission computed tomography combined with conventional computed tomography 10 months post-TAA showed increased uptake at the medial and lateral talo-malleolar area. (*D*) Weight-bearing ankle AP view shows cleared gutters after gutter debridement.

Our preference for gutter debridement is an open approach. The polyethylene is removed so that the talus may be adequately mobilized. Both gutters are examined and debrided, however special attention is paid to the symptomatic side. In cases of lateral gutter debridement, often the medial aspect of the fibula requires partial resection. If the debridement is closer to the tip of the fibula, a separate lateral incision may be necessary. In cases of medial gutter impingement, the anteromedial aspect of the talus is debrided, as well as the lateral aspect of the medial malleolus (**Fig. 3**). A prophylactic screw is often placed in the medial malleolus if there is not one there already because medial gutter impingement can be difficult to differentiate from medial distal tibial stress reaction after TAA. Trial polyethylene inserts are then used to determine if upsizing the polyethylene is possible. Ideally, a larger polyethylene will help distract the gutters assuming motion at the ankle is not sacrificed. Any additional procedures to realign the ankle and foot can be done at the same time as the gutter debridement to optimize postoperative outcomes.

OUTCOMES OF REOPERATION FOR GUTTER IMPINGEMENT

Although many clinical follow-up studies have reported the number of patients experiencing gutter impingement pain or undergoing gutter debridement as a subsequent surgery, only a few studies have documented the outcomes of reoperations due to gutter impingement. Kurup and colleagues made one of the earliest reports on the outcomes of gutter debridement after TAA.[14] They reported on the outcomes of reoperations for 4 patients (out of 34 total TAA patients) with medial impingement symptoms. Two of these patients underwent medial gutter debridement (1 arthroscopically and 1 through an open procedure), whereas the other 2 underwent decompression of the posterior tibial tendon. All patients were symptom-free after the reoperation, with a minimum follow-up of 6 months.

Shirzad and colleagues described an arthroscopic technique to resect bony and soft-tissue impingement around the ankle joint, including the medial and lateral

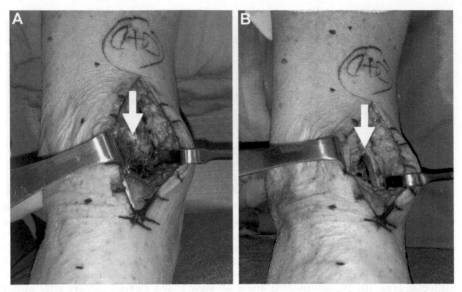

Fig. 3. Intraoperative images of a patient who underwent medial gutter debridement following TAA. (*A*) Before the gutter debridement, almost no space is visible between the talar implant and medial malleolus due to bony overgrowth (*arrow*). (*B*) After gutter debridement, a clear space is visible between the implant and medial malleolus (*arrow*).

gutters.[44] They reported a decrease in pain in 11 patients but did not report objective patient-reported outcome scores.

Richardson and colleagues reported the outcomes of an arthroscopic gutter debridement procedure in 20 patients, with 18 of them having sufficient follow-up to assess the success of the procedure.[21] Of the 20 patients, 80% (16 patients) reported an initial resolution of their pain following the procedure. However, among the 4 patients with poor outcomes, 1 had developed talar component subsidence and 2 were planned for repeat arthroscopy, whereas 1 was planned for open arthrotomy at the time of the report. What was striking from their report was that of the 16 patients who initially resolved their symptoms, 6 (37.5%) later developed recurrent symptoms and required further intervention, such as 3 open arthrotomies, 2 distal fibular resections, and 1 distal medial malleolar resection.

Kim and colleagues investigated the outcomes of arthroscopic debridement in patients who experienced residual pain after mobile-bearing TAA.[24] Among the 7 patients (5.8% of 120 TAAs) who underwent arthroscopic debridement, scar tissue with associated synovitis was observed, causing anterior impingement as well as impingement in both medial and lateral gutters. In contrast to studies by Shirzad and colleagues and Richardson and colleagues, the researchers used a harness for ankle distraction. Following debridement, the median pain visual analog scale (VAS) scores significantly decreased from 7 to 3 ($P < .001$), and all but one patient were satisfied with the outcome. In the mean follow-up period of 40 months, there was no significant difference in the VAS and American Orthopedic Foot and Ankle Society ankle-hindfoot score between patients who underwent arthroscopic debridement and those who did not ($P = .148$).

Schuberth and colleagues presented the largest retrospective series of 489 TAAs using 4 different systems and determined that symptomatic gutter disease occurred in 34 (7%) cases at a mean follow-up of 68 months.[22] Of the 34 patients, 30 met the

12-month follow-up criteria and all reported a subjective reduction in preoperative symptoms at the final clinical follow-up. On the postoperative questionnaire, only 9 of 30 patients (30%) reported no recurrence of pain, whereas 21 patients (70%) reported persistent pain even after the debridement, with an average VAS pain score of 3.5. Additionally, 60% (18 out of 30) of patients reported persistent limitations after gutter debridement.

Although there are few studies on the long-term follow-up after reoperation due to gutter impingement, a study by Kim and colleagues compared the minimum 5-year outcomes between patients who had reoperation due to gutter impingement (n = 11) and those without (n = 60) after receiving Salto Talaris TAA using the Foot and Ankle Outcome Score (FAOS).[20] The mean time to reoperation was 30.5 months. The results showed that although all patients reported improvement in their symptoms after reoperation, the FAOS scores at the final follow-up were significantly lower in the group that underwent gutter debridement. Additionally, the group with gutter impingement showed less improvement in the Pain, Symptoms, and Quality of Life subscales compared with the group without reoperation. However, there were no differences in the coronal and sagittal implant alignment as seen on plain radiographs.

The review of earlier studies reveals some similarities in that gutter debridement is effective in alleviating impingement symptoms in the shorter term but it still has a relatively high recurrence rate, residual pain, and reduced functional performance in the longer term. This suggests that gutter impingement may be a more complicated condition than previously understood, and that gutter debridement alone may not be a sufficient solution for some patients. Ideally, all efforts must be made to avoid gutter impingement at the time of the initial surgery, with special attention to appropriate alignment of the implant including the axial plane, appropriate sizing of the components, and balancing the foot underneath the ankle.

Most studies that reported gutter impingement were actually based on plain radiographs, which can show the coronal and sagittal alignment of the implant. As Najefi and colleagues suggested,[39] the axial plane alignment of the implant may play an important role in the development of gutter impingement symptoms. Additionally, axial malrotation may be associated with altered kinematics of the ankle joint, which may explain the worse FAOS score in the gutter debridement group in the medium-term in the study by Kim and colleagues.[20] The use of WBCT will be of great help in identifying this, and at the same time, gutter impingement patients can be assessed for any cyst formation, subsidence, or heterotopic ossification that is not readily identifiable on plain radiographs. As Mason and colleagues suggested,[43] the use of SPECT-CT can also be helpful in identifying the causes of gutter impingement symptoms, if accessible.

Another factor that is missing in earlier evaluations of gutter impingement patients is hindfoot and lower limb alignment assessment. As stated above, hindfoot or lower limb mechanical axis may affect the development of gutter impingement[34–36] but no study has yet assessed them. We believe that correction of malalignment at the foot, hindfoot, or even at the distal tibia should be considered to warrant a longer term resolution of gutter impingement symptoms.

SUMMARY

Gutter impingement is a relatively common complication of TAA that often leads to subsequent surgery. Although gutter debridement is frequently performed to resolve patient symptoms, surgeons should be aware that gutter impingement can be more than inadequate debridement at the time of initial surgery. Previous assessments of gutter impingement have largely been based on coronal plane x-rays but an understanding of this complication in 3 dimensions using advanced imaging modalities such as WBCT may be helpful. Simultaneously exploring possible causes outside the ankle joint, such as foot, hindfoot, or lower limb alignment, may help determine the underlying causes of gutter impingement and optimize reoperation outcomes.

CLINICS CARE POINTS

- Careful selection of the implant size is necessary to minimize risk for gutter impingement. Upsizing the polyethylene insert is beneficial as long as motion is not sacrificed.
- Perform a thorough gutter debridement to decrease the risk of postoperative gutter impingement.
- Be mindful of the axial rotation of the implant. Internal rotation of the components may increase the likelihood of medial gutter impingement postoperatively. When planning for the rotational alignment of the implant, a preoperative weight bearing CT is helpful.
- SPECT-CT and/or WBCT can help confirm the diagnosis of gutter impingement postoperatively.

CONFLICT OF INTEREST

J. Kim: Nothing to disclose. C. Demetracopoulos: American Orthopedic Foot and Ankle Society: Board or committee member. Exactech, Inc: IP royalties; Paid consultant; Paid presenter or speaker. In2Bones: IP royalties; Paid consultant Medshape: Paid consultant. RTI Surgical: Paid consultant. Wolters Kluwer Health - Lippincott Williams & Wilkins: Publishing royalties, financial or material support.

REFERENCES

1. Randsborg P-H, Jiang H, Mao J, et al. Two-year revision rates in total ankle replacement versus ankle arthrodesis: a population-based propensity-score-matched comparison from new York state and california. JBJS Open Access 2022;7(2):e21.
2. Gougoulias NE, Khanna A, Maffulli N. History and evolution in total ankle arthroplasty. Br Med Bull 2009;89(1):111–51.
3. Haddad S, Coetzee J, Estok R, et al. Intermediate and long-term outcomes of total ankle arthroplasty and ankle arthrodesis: a systematic review of the literature. JBJS 2007;89(9):1899–905.
4. Day J, Kim J, O'Malley MJ, et al. Radiographic and clinical outcomes of the Salto Talaris total ankle arthroplasty. Foot Ankle Int 2020;41(12):1519–28.
5. SooHoo NF, Zingmond DS, Ko CY. Comparison of reoperation rates following ankle arthrodesis and total ankle arthroplasty. JBJS 2007;89(10):2143–9.
6. Hofmann KJ, Shabin ZM, Ferkel E, et al. Salto Talaris total ankle arthroplasty: clinical results at a mean of 5.2 years in 78 patients treated by a single surgeon. JBJS 2016;98(24):2036–46.
7. Spirt AA, Assal M, Hansen ST Jr. Complications and failure after total ankle arthroplasty. JBJS 2004;86(6):1172–8.
8. Younger AS, Glazebrook M, Veljkovic A, et al. A coding system for reoperations following total ankle replacement and ankle arthrodesis. Foot Ankle Int 2016; 37(11):1157–64.

9. Kim J, Gagne OJ, Rajan L, et al. Clinical outcomes of the lateral trabecular metal total ankle replacement at a 5-year minimum follow-up. Foot & Ankle Specialist; 2022:19386400221139525.

10. Gagne OJ, Day J, Kim J, et al. Midterm survivorship of the INBONE II total ankle arthroplasty. Foot Ankle Int 2022;43(5):628–36.

11. Rajan L, Kim J, Cronin S, et al. Retrospective comparison of midterm survivorship, radiographic, and clinical outcomes of the INBONE II and Salto Talaris total ankle arthroplasty systems. Foot Ankle Int 2022;43(11):1419–23.

12. Kim J, Rajan L, Bitar R, et al. Early radiographic and clinical outcomes of a novel, fixed-bearing fourth-generation total ankle replacement system. Foot Ankle Int 2022;43(11):1424–33.

13. Shih C-L, Chen S-J, Huang P-J. Clinical outcomes of total ankle arthroplasty versus ankle arthrodesis for the treatment of end-stage ankle arthritis in the last decade: a systematic review and meta-analysis. J Foot Ankle Surg 2020;59(5): 1032–9.

14. Kurup HV, Taylor GR. Medial impingement after ankle replacement. Int Orthop 2008;32:243–6.

15. Hintermann B, Valderrabano V, Dereymaeker G, et al. The HINTEGRA ankle: rationale and short-term results of 122 consecutive ankles. Clin Orthop Relat Res (1976-2007) 2004;424:57–68.

16. Rippstein PF, Huber M, Coetzee JC, et al. Total ankle replacement with use of a new three-component implant. JBJS 2011;93(15):1426–35.

17. Easley ME, Adams SB Jr, Hembree WC, et al. Results of total ankle arthroplasty. JBJS 2011;93(15):1455–68.

18. Mann JA, Mann RA, Horton E. STAR™ ankle: long-term results. Foot Ankle Int 2011;32(5):473–84.

19. Hermus J, Voesenek J, van Gansewinkel E, et al. Complications following total ankle arthroplasty: a systematic literature review and meta-analysis. Foot Ankle Surg 2022. https://doi.org/10.1016/j.fas.2022.07.004.

20. Kim J, Rajan L, Fuller R, et al. Mid-term functional outcomes following reoperation after total ankle arthroplasty: A retrospective cohort study. Foot Ankle Surg 2022; 28(8):1463–7.

21. Richardson AB, DeOrio JK, Parekh SG. Arthroscopic debridement: effective treatment for impingement after total ankle arthroplasty. Current reviews in musculoskeletal medicine 2012;5:171–5.

22. Schuberth JM, Babu NS, Richey JM, et al. Gutter impingement after total ankle arthroplasty. Foot Ankle Int 2013;34(3):329–37.

23. Schuberth JM, Wood DA, Christensen JC. Gutter impingement in total ankle arthroplasty. Foot Ankle Spec 2016;9(2):145–58.

24. Kim B, Choi W, Kim J, et al. Residual pain due to soft-tissue impingement after uncomplicated total ankle replacement. The Bone & Joint Journal 2013;95(3): 378–83.

25. Gurbani A, Demetracopoulos C, O'Malley M, et al. Correlation of single-photon emission computed tomography results with clinical and intraoperative findings in painful total ankle replacement. Foot Ankle Int 2020;41(6):639–46.

26. Gross CE, Palanca AA, DeOrio JK. Design rationale for total ankle arthroplasty systems: an update. JAAOS-Journal of the American Academy of Orthopaedic Surgeons. 2018;26(10):353–9.

27. Brodsky J, Kane J, Coleman S, et al. Abnormalities of gait caused by ankle arthritis are improved by ankle arthrodesis. The bone & joint journal 2016; 98(10):1369–75.

28. Valderrabano V, Nigg BM, von Tscharner V, et al. Gait analysis in ankle osteoarthritis and total ankle replacement. Clin BioMech 2007;22(8):894–904.
29. Kim J-B, Yi Y, Kim J-Y, et al. Weight-bearing computed tomography findings in varus ankle osteoarthritis: abnormal internal rotation of the talus in the axial plane. Skeletal Radiol 2017;46:1071–80.
30. Easley ME, Vertullo CJ, Urban CW, et al. Total ankle arthroplasty. JAAOS-Journal of the American Academy of Orthopaedic Surgeons. 2002;10(3):157–67.
31. Cenni F, Leardini A, Belvedere C, et al. Kinematics of the three components of a total ankle replacement: in vivo fluoroscopic analysis. Foot Ankle Int 2012;33(4): 290–300.
32. Leszko F, Komistek RD, Mahfouz MR, et al. In vivo kinematics of the Salto total ankle prosthesis. Foot Ankle Int 2008;29(11):1117–25.
33. Nunley JA, Adams SB, Easley ME, et al. Prospective randomized trial comparing mobile-bearing and fixed-bearing total ankle replacement. Foot Ankle Int 2019; 40(11):1239–48.
34. Barg A, Suter T, Zwicky L, et al. Medial pain syndrome in patients with total ankle replacement. Orthopä 2011;40:991–9.
35. Bevernage BD, Deleu P-A, Kurup HV, et al. Management of Painful Malleolar Gutters After Total Ankle Replacement. Primary and revision total ankle replacement: evidence-based surgical management. 2016:223-230.
36. Yi Y, Cho J-H, Kim J-B, et al. Change in talar translation in the coronal plane after mobile-bearing total ankle replacement and its association with lower-limb and hindfoot alignment. JBJS 2017;99(4):e13.
37. Gagné OJ, Penner M, Wing K, et al. Reoperation profile of lateral vs anterior approach ankle arthroplasty. Foot Ankle Int 2020;41(7):834–8.
38. Cerrato R, Myerson MS. Total ankle replacement: the Agility LP prosthesis. Foot Ankle Clin 2008;13(3):485–94.
39. Najefi A-A, Ghani Y, Goldberg A. Role of rotation in total ankle replacement. Foot Ankle Int 2019;40(12):1358–67.
40. Saito GH, Sturnick DR, Ellis SJ, et al. Influence of tibial component position on altered kinematics following total ankle arthroplasty during simulated gait. Foot Ankle Int 2019;40(8):873–9.
41. Kim BS, Lee JW. Arthroscopic debridement for soft-tissue impingement after total ankle replacement. Primary and revision total ankle replacement: evidence-based surgical management. 2016:211-215.
42. Devos Bevernage B, Deleu P-A, Birch I, et al. Arthroscopic debridement after total ankle arthroplasty. Foot Ankle Int 2016;37(2):142–9.
43. Mason LW, Wyatt J, Butcher C, et al. Single-photon-emission computed tomography in painful total ankle replacements. Foot Ankle Int 2015;36(6):635–40. https://doi.org/10.1177/1071100715573050.
44. Shirzad K, Viens NA, DeOrio JK. Arthroscopic treatment of impingement after total ankle arthroplasty: technique tip. Foot Ankle Int 2011;32(7):727–9. https://doi.org/10.3113/fai.2011.0727.

Outcomes of Total Ankle Arthroplasty After Periprosthetic Cyst Curettage and Bone Grafting

Paulo N.F. Ferrao, MBChB (Pret), FCS Ortho (SA)[a,b,*],
Nikiforos P. Saragas, FCS (SA) Ortho, PhD (Wits)[a,b],
Jaco J. Naude, FC Ortho (SA), MMed Orth (Pret)[a,c]

KEYWORDS

- Total ankle arthroplasty • Periprosthetic cysts • Bone grafting • Osteolysis

KEY POINTS

- Total ankle arthroplasty has become a popular and viable management option for end-stage ankle arthritis.
- Periprosthetic osteolysis is a common cause for reoperation and revision surgery.
- Osteolytic bone cysts develop as a response to inflammatory mediated osteoclastic bone resorption.
- A computed tomographic scan with metal subtraction should be done in all suspected cyst cases to confirm location, quantify lesion size, and aid in surgical planning when indicated.
- Curettage and bone grafting of asymptomatic large periprosthetic cysts can be beneficial in preventing implant displacement and failure, thereby increasing the implant survival and functional outcomes.

INTRODUCTION

Osteoarthritis (OA) of the ankle is a progressive destructive disease of the joint that results in severe pain and reduced joint motion leading to limited activities of daily living and ultimately decreased quality of life. This decrease in quality of life has been found to be equivalent to end-stage renal disease or congestive cardiac failure.[1–3] Total ankle arthroplasty (TAA) has become a popular and accepted management option

[a] The Orthopaedic Foot & Ankle Unit, Netcare Linksfield Hospital, 303 Linksfield Medical Centre, 24 12th Avenue, Linksfield West, 2192, South Africa; [b] Department of Orthopaedic Surgery, University of the Witwatersrand, 7 York Road, Parktown, Johannesburg, 2193, South Africa; [c] Life Wilgers Hospital, Denneboom road, Wilgers ext 14, Pretoria, 0040, South Africa
* Corresponding author. 303 Linksfield medical centre, 24 12th avenue, Linksfield West, 2192, South Africa.
E-mail address: paulo@cybersmart.co.za

Foot Ankle Clin N Am 29 (2024) 123–143
https://doi.org/10.1016/j.fcl.2023.08.006
1083-7515/24/© 2023 Elsevier Inc. All rights reserved.

for ankle OA owing to the advancement of implants (third and fourth generation), improved surgical techniques, and refined indications.

TAA survival rates using modern day implants have improved to 70% to 100% at 5 years and 71% to 77% at 10 years' follow-up.[4] Aseptic loosening is reported as the most common cause for implant failure, accounting for 28% to 55% of TAA revision cases.[5–9] Periprosthetic cysts are one of the causes of aseptic loosening. Periprosthetic cysts are defined as lucencies with absent osseous trabecula and sclerotic borders at the bone-implant interface.[10] The incidence of periprosthetic cysts has been reported to be as high as 95% in TAA at mid- and long-term follow-up, which is significantly higher than after hip and knee arthroplasty.[11–24] Day and colleagues[25] and Bonnin and colleagues[12] reported incidences of 21.2% and 22.3%, respectively, of cysts over the size of 5 mm with the Salto Talaris prosthesis (Smith & Nephew, Memphis, TN). Arcangelo and colleagues[26] reported in a systematic review that the timing to diagnosis of periprosthetic cysts ranges from 6 to 89 months after TAA. The significance of these cysts with regard to implant failure is uncertain at this stage, as they vary in cause, size, and location.

Most periprosthetic cysts identified during follow-up are asymptomatic but have the potential to enlarge, resulting in mechanical failure with a negative impact on implant survival.[5,11,27,28] The indications and management of periprosthetic cysts are challenging, as there is limited literature available to guide surgeons. One needs to weigh the risk of cyst progression with potential implant failure against the risk of having a second surgery.

TYPES OF CYSTS

Two types of cysts have been identified in patients with TAA.

Degenerative Bone Cysts

These are subchondral bone cysts that develop as part of the disease process in joint arthritis. The pathophysiology of these cysts begins with attrition of the cartilage exposing the underlying subchondral bone.[29] Two theories have been described for the formation of the subchondral cysts.

The "synovial fluid intrusion theory"
The subchondral bone fails under load, allowing synovial fluid to enter the cancellous bone under pressure, forming cysts.[30–32]

The "bone contusion theory"
The exposed subchondral bone gets abnormally loaded, causing excessive mechanical stress, which results in surrounding edema.[30,32,33] This stress response activates osteoblasts, inflammatory cytokines, and proteinases, causing bone resorption. Crema and colleagues[30,34] in a longitudinal MRI study demonstrated that this bone marrow edema results in cyst formation in areas of cartilage attrition.

Najefi and colleagues[29] reported that 78% of patients with ankle OA would have residual degenerative bone cysts after bone resection for TAA, of which 33% were greater than 5 mm in size. Of note, 69% of cysts were in the medial and lateral malleoli and thus not in contact with the implants. Interestingly, the investigators noted that 60% of these cysts were not apparent on plain radiographs. The natural history of these cysts with regard to progression is unknown and requires further research.

Osteolytic Bone Cysts

These cysts develop as a response to macrophage-activated osteoclastic bone resorption.[29] This is the more common type of cyst associated with implant failure.

The pathophysiology of periprosthetic osteolytic cysts is not fully understood, but numerous etiologic factors have been described. These factors are either mechanical or biological processes, which often go hand in hand[35] (**Table 1**).

Implant-related factors

Nonanatomic implant designs have complex multidirectional motion that results in higher mechanical interfacial shearing stress.[1,5,26,36] This in turn results in abnormal loading and increased wear patterns resulting in microdebris formation.

Mobile bearing surfaces have the benefit of a conforming articulation with superior kinematics but result in smaller, granular particles from normal wear. Mobile bearing implants also have 2 articulating surfaces that could increase the concentration of wear particles. Fixed bearing surfaces have a harsher wear pattern consisting of delamination and pitting, which results in larger-sized debris particles.[26,37–42] Cottrino and colleagues[26,43] reported that wear particles need to be smaller than 50 μm to be phagocytosed by macrophages and thereby inducing an inflammatory response. This could explain why mobile bearing implants result in more osteolytic cysts despite having better kinematics.

Implant coating with hydroxyapatite (HA) has been implicated with a higher incidence of osteolytic cysts. Singh and colleagues[44] reported that HA coating is a contributing factor to ballooning osteolysis in patients with TAA. Khademi and colleagues[3] reported the histologic findings of periprosthetic cyst contents in patients with a Hintegra prosthesis (Newdeal, Lyon, France; Integra Lifesciences, Plainsboro, NJ) and identified HA in all specimens (**Fig. 1**).

Nonstemmed tibial implants have been reported to have a higher incidence of cysts, most likely owing to the implant being less stable with increased motion at the implant-bone interface. However, when periprosthetic cysts develop with stemmed tibial implants, they are reported to be larger in size and required more revision surgeries. These cysts are thought to develop because of stress shielding from the stem.[26]

Incomplete coverage of resected bony surfaces by the implants have been implicated with cyst formation. This occurs most commonly around the talar neck, medial and lateral sides of the tibia, exposing the bare bone to the synovial fluid, which is under pressure. This has been described as the "effective joint concept" by which the pressurized synovial fluid in a small joint causes cyst formation.[45–47]

The Ankle Evolutive System (AES) ankle replacement was a prime example of an implant with inherent design flaws. Besse and colleagues[11] reported at the 2-year follow-up that 62% and 43% of cases had tibial and talar osteolytic cysts, respectively. Kohonen and colleagues[10] reported the management of periprosthetic cysts

Table 1 Possible etiologic factors in the development of periprosthetic bone cysts	
Etiologic Factors of Osteolysis	
Implant-related factors	Nonanatomic designs Mobile bearing surfaces Implant coating (HA) Nonstemmed tibial implants Incomplete coverage of resected bony surfaces
Surgical technique	Implant malalignment Lower limb malalignment
Third body concept	Inflammatory response to PE, metal, and HA wear particles
Micromotion	Implant motion of >150 μm at bone interface

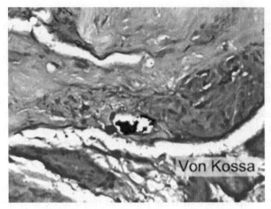

Fig. 1. Von Kossa staining of periprosthetic osteolytic cyst content showing the presence of HA.

with a failure rate of 68%. Of note, 91% of their patients had the AES prosthesis. The high failure rate was most probably because of the inherent design flaws of the prosthesis. The AES prosthesis was ultimately withdrawn from the market in 2008 because of the excessively high rate of periprosthetic cyst formation.

Surgical technique

When compared with total knee and hip replacements, a malpositioned TAA is less forgiving with resultant abnormal loading and sheer stress. This then leads to bone edema and increased wear particles formation, both of which result in osteolysis.[11,26,46,48,49] In the literature, increased contact pressures and higher rates of subsidence have been reported with malalignment of the prosthesis, especially of the talar component.[50–53] It is critical that the surgeon be meticulous with the surgical technique and implant alignment.[2,25,35,49,54]

Third body mediated inflammatory response

Wear particles of polyethylene (PE), metal, and HA have been identified in periprosthetic cyst tissue.[3,36,55–57] Phagocytoses of these wear particles by the macrophages cause a release of proinflammatory cytokines, including tumor necrosis factor-α, interleukin-1 (IL-1), and IL-6, which lead to bone lysis and bone resorption by inhibiting osteoblast activity and activating osteoclast activity.[1,24,43,55,57,58] As mentioned previously, the particles size (<50 μm) and concentration will determine the biological response by the host. It has been suggested that some hosts are genetically more sensitive to wear particles and have been termed "implant looseners."[1,59]

Micromotion

Micromotion is submillimeter movement between the prosthesis and bone interface.[58] The ideal amount of micromotion for bony ingrowth has been reported to be less than 150 μm. Micromotion of more than 150 μm causes fibrous ingrowth, which allows for a void at the implant-bone interface. This allows for high-pressure synovial fluid and wear particles to infiltrate into the void, which leads to inflammatory cell mediated bone lysis.[1,58,60,61] McInnes and colleagues[62] reported that the Agility ankle prosthesis (DePuy Synthes Orthopedics, Warsaw, IN, USA) has more micromotion as compared with the STAR ankle prosthesis (Stryker, Kalamazoo, MI), which could account for the increased incidence of aseptic loosening with the Agility prosthesis.

Yoon and colleagues[24] defined periprosthetic cysts as being early-onset and late-onset cysts. Any periprosthetic cysts identified within 1 year of the primary procedure were defined as early-onset cysts. They reported that only 9.5% of early-onset cysts showed progression in size, whereas 50% of late-onset cysts showed progression in size during follow-up. Najefi and colleagues[29] reported that the early-onset cysts are often residual preoperative degenerative bone cysts. It has been suggested that these degenerative bone cysts are less likely to progress. Further research is required regarding evolution and effects of these degenerative bone cysts. Knecht and colleagues[63] concluded that late-onset cysts are due to true inflammatory bone loss.

SPECIAL INVESTIGATIONS
Radiographs

Weight-bearing radiographs of the ankle are routine when following up patients with a TAA. The radiographs are used to assess implant alignment and look for changes in implant position and the presence of periprosthetic cysts. A gap of less than 2 mm at the bone-implant interface is considered to be a radiolucency, whereas osteolytic cysts are defined as nonlinear lytic lesions measuring 2 mm or greater in width[24] (**Fig. 2**). Besse and colleagues[11] described Gruen-like zones in the tibia and talus to document cyst location and size. Using zones will standardize the reporting of cyst location for documenting and research purposes[3,11,25,64] (**Fig. 3**). The current literature has revealed that radiographs have a low sensitivity for identifying osteolytic cysts. The reason for this is that the distal tibia has a high cortical density relative to the cancellous bone, making the metaphyseal cysts difficult to visualize on radiographs, and second, the cysts can be obscured by the metal implant itself.[24] Hanna and colleagues[14] reported that radiographs only detected 52% of cysts less than 200 mm^2 as compared with computed tomography (CT) scans. Yoon and colleagues[24] reported that the sensitivity of radiographs was only 53% and 50% for detecting osteolytic cysts of any size and less than 100 mm^2, respectively. As radiographs are 2 dimensional, they are inaccurate in quantifying the true size of periprosthetic cysts.

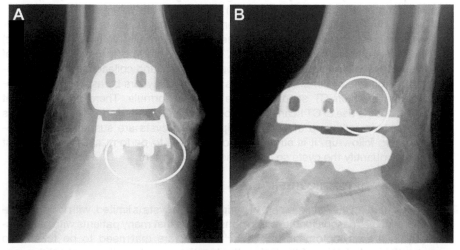

Fig. 2. (A) Anteroposterior weight-bearing radiograph of the ankle with a periprosthetic cyst (demarcated by the *yellow circle*) under the talus. (B) Oblique weight-bearing radiograph of the ankle with a periprosthetic cyst (demarcated by the *yellow circle*) in the tibia.

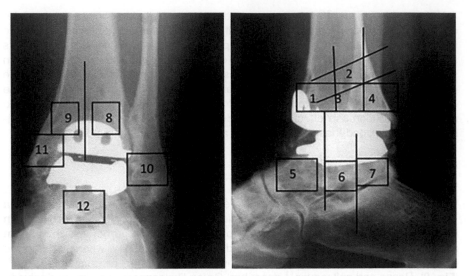

Fig. 3. Gruen-like zones in the tibia and talus for documenting size and location of periprosthetic cysts.

Computed Tomography Scans

CT scan with metal-artifact suppression has become the preferred investigation for detecting and accurately measuring the size of periprosthetic cysts.[26] Studies have reported that up to 87% of lesions detected on CT scans had initial inaccurate radiographic interpretations.[10,24,29,64–66] Najefi and colleagues[29] reported on 31 patients that had cysts identified on radiographs. Only 7 patients had all the cysts detected on radiographs after reviewing the CT scans. Hanna and colleagues[14] noted that cysts on CT scan were 3 times larger as compared with measurements on corresponding radiographs, with 87% of cysts being inaccurately reported on radiographs. Initial studies quantified cyst size by measuring the longest dimension in only 2 planes, thus reporting on the area (2 dimensional) rather than the volume of the cysts.[14,24] The benefit of CT scan is that all 3 dimensions can be assessed. Gross and colleagues[67] calculated cyst volume using the ellipsoid formula (Volume $= 4/3\pi*x*y*z$) by taking measurements in all 3 axes (**Fig. 4**). This is a far more accurate method of quantifying cyst volume and should be adopted. Naude and colleagues[68] recently reported the outcome of periprosthetic cysts grafting at 3 years by assessing incorporation of the graft on CT scan using the ellipsoid formula. There are no current guidelines, but the use of CT scans should be considered part of special investigations during long-term follow-up of TAA. If periprosthetic cysts are suspected on radiographs during follow-up, it is strongly recommended to perform a CT scan to best localize and quantify the cysts so as to guide management.

MANAGEMENT OF PERIPROSTHETIC CYSTS

Literature regarding the management of periprosthetic cysts is limited, with varying strategies. One of the reasons for the lack in consensus is that many patients with periprosthetic cysts are asymptomatic.[5,11,25,27,28,69,70] Factors that need to be taken into consideration include size of the lesion, the location, growth pattern, patients' symptoms, and the impact on the implant and surrounding bone. Although mostly asymptomatic, these cysts can enlarge and ultimately cause mechanical failure with a negative

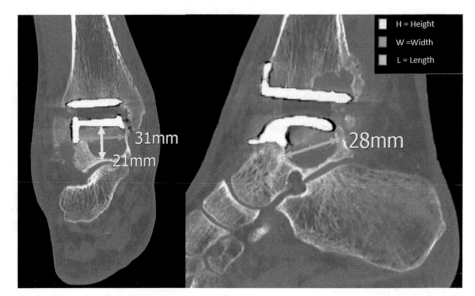

Fig. 4. Coronal and sagittal CT scan cuts of a talar periprosthetic cysts used to calculate the volume using the ellipsoid formula: $4/3\pi*H*W*L$.

consequence for implant survival. Currently there are no clear guidelines. From the available literature, suggested indications are the following:

1. Periprosthetic cysts causing pain
2. Rapid progression in cyst size
3. Cysts occupying more than one-third of the bone-implant interface
4. Massive area of osteolysis, which could result in a stress fracture or destabilize the implant[10,16,24,26,58,67,68,71,72]

The treatment of asymptomatic cysts is challenging, as the risk of cyst progression and implant failure must be compared with the risk of a second surgery.[35] Recent studies have shown the advantages of more aggressive operative management of asymptomatic periprosthetic cysts.[12,16,26,71,73] Treatment can be divided into monitoring for cyst progression, curettage and bone grafting, revision of TAA, or conversion to an arthrodesis (ankle or tibiotalocalcaneal).

Monitoring for Cyst Progression

Smaller asymptomatic cysts should be managed conservatively with diligent follow-up, including a CT scan to quantify cyst size on an annual basis. Definition of a small cyst varies from 2 mm to 10 mm in the literature.[12,35,68] Should the patient become symptomatic at any stage, surgical management is indicated. Naude and colleagues[68] demonstrated that cysts with a volume less than 1.75 cm^3 had very little progression, whereas cysts with this volume or greater increased significantly in size over the 3-year follow-up period.

Curettage and Bone Grafting of Cyst

This management is indicated in patients meeting the following criteria[12,16,35,57,67,71,74]:

a. Symptomatic cysts

b. Asymptomatic cysts rapidly progressing in size
c. Asymptomatic cysts 10 to 15 mm or larger in all axes on CT scan
d. Contained cysts with cortical integrity
e. Stable and well-aligned implants

Gross and colleagues[67] and Naude and colleagues[68] reported that bone grafting of periprosthetic cysts without revision of the prosthesis was effective and may increase implant survivorship. Bone grafting with successful incorporation can possibly result in stability of the implant and decrease cyst progression and revision rates.

Revision of Total Ankle Arthroplasty

Numerous TAA systems have developed revision systems for the management of unstable, malaligned, or subsided components. Because of the functional limitations, complexity, and high complication rate of arthrodesis after a failed TAA, revision TAA has gained in popularity. Bone grafting of the cysts is often required when doing a revision TAA. Criteria for revision TAR include the following[35,58]:

a. Large uncontained cysts
b. Unstable or malaligned TAA
c. Adequate bone stock
d. Surgeon technical know how

Arthrodesis

Arthrodesis is challenging due to the significant defect after TAA with massive osteolysis. Often a structural tricortical autograft, femoral head allograft, or custom titanium cage is required with varying rates of successful fusion reported in the literature.[75–77] Rates of nonunion in the literature after conversion of a failed TAA to arthrodesis vary from 11% to 42%.[29,78–83]

The criteria for arthrodesis are as follows[35]:

a. Inadequate bone stock
b. Significant talar bone loss
c. Poor-quality anterior soft tissue

Types of bone graft and substitutes used

a. *Autogenous bone graft* is readily available and the gold standard with regard to bone grafting. The harvesting of autogenous bone graft does come with the risk of comorbidities and thus is avoided by some surgeons. Common donor sites are the iliac crest, proximal and distal tibia, and the calcaneus. The authors have found the proximal tibia to supply sufficient autogenous bone, using an 8-mm trephine, for most cysts that they have treated with minimal comorbidities. If a cyst requires excessive amounts of bone graft, then they will harvest from the iliac crest. Most the available literature reports using autogenous bone graft.[12,24,68,83–86]
b. *Allograft bone chips* eliminate the morbidities associated with harvesting autogenous bone. Gross and colleagues[67] reported a large case series using allograft bone chips with a 91% success rate at 2 years, which then dropped to 60% at 4 years. It is questionable whether this drop in success is related to the use of allograft. Kohonen and colleagues[16] used allograft bone in 85% of their cases with poor results. The authors cannot deduce much from these results, as 90% of the implants were AES. Therefore, the poor results in this study may be related to the implant itself rather than the allograft bone.

c. *Polymethylmethacrylate cement* has been used in a small number of cases for very large lesions.[67] Because the cement has no biological properties and merely serves as a filler and structural support, it is not routinely recommended.
d. *Calcium phosphate filler* was reported on by Gross and colleagues[67] in 4 patients with periprosthetic bone cysts. Of the cases, 75% required reoperation, and thus, calcium phosphate as a bone graft substitute is not recommended.

Use of bone supplements

Mesenchymal stem cells, platelet-rich plasma, recombinant human bone morphogenic proteins (BMP), and demineralized bone matrix (DBM) have all been used as adjuncts in the literature.[67,68] The case numbers are too low to draw any conclusion regarding the effectiveness of bone supplements. The authors routinely supplement the bone graft with a DBM containing BMPs. This serves 2 purposes: It increases the volume of the bone graft, and, it is hoped, adds osteoinductive properties. If these are available, it would be recommended to use them.

THE AUTHORS' MANAGEMENT PROTOCOL
Degenerative Bone Cysts

These are usually the early periprosthetic cysts that are identified within the first 2 years after TAA. Najefi and colleagues[29] reported that many of these cysts occur in the

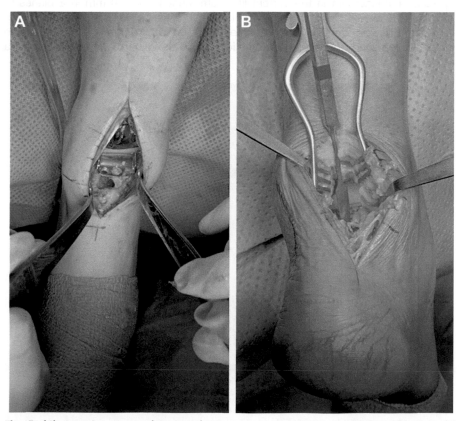

Fig. 5. (*A*) Anterior approach using the previous incision to an anterior talar cyst. (*B*) Posterolateral approach to a posterior talar cyst.

medial and lateral malleoli, which could result in fracture if the cysts were to expand. Currently, there are no data regarding the natural evolution of these cysts as to whether they enlarge or remain benign. The authors will routinely bone graft any large degenerative cysts found at the bone-implant interface at the time of primary surgery or if identified on preoperative radiographs. Degenerative cysts in the malleoli are monitored, and if expansile, are bone grafted to prevent possible fractures. Najefi and colleagues[29] have recommended routine preoperative CT scan of the ankle in patients undergoing a TAA, so as to better identify these degenerative cysts and manage them accordingly at the time of primary surgery. Further research regarding the natural evolution and effect of these degenerative cysts is required.

Osteolytic Bone Cysts

All patients with TAA are followed up on an annual basis with routine weight-bearing ankle radiographs. Even though careful clinical examination will help differentiate the cause for pain, early osteolysis is not always accompanied by pain or loss of function. In a recent publication regarding periprosthetic cysts, 88% of patients were asymptomatic.[68] If periprosthetic cysts are identified on radiographs, a CT scan with metal suppression is performed to better define the cyst with regard to location and size. Because of the limited available literature, no consensus has been achieved regarding an absolute cyst size, which requires bone grafting. The suggested size for operative management in the current literature ranges from 10 mm in 2 planes to 15 mm in 3 planes.[16,17,24,26,58,67,71,84] The authors use a volume of greater than 1.75 cm^3 (Ellipsoid formula), which equates to a cyst with 15 mm in all 3 axes, as an indication for bone grafting asymptomatic cysts. This value of 15 mm is merely a

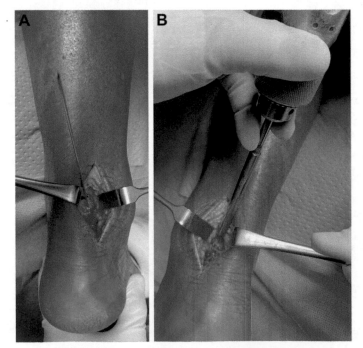

Fig. 6. (*A*) The cyst is identified and marked using a K-wire under fluoroscopy. (*B*) A bony window is opened into the cyst by using an 8-mm trephine over the K-wire as a guide.

guideline, similar to what was used by Lundeen and colleagues.[84] Further large-volume multicenter studies will be needed to define the exact size of the periprosthetic cyst that should be bone grafted. The cyst also needs to be contained with no cortical lysis, and the implant must be well aligned and stable. All symptomatic cysts are bone grafted routinely. Periprosthetic bone cysts smaller than 1.75 cm^3 are monitored on an annual basis using CT scan imaging.[68]

Surgical technique

Patients are placed supine or prone depending on the cyst location. An above-knee tourniquet can be used. Anterior cysts are approached through the previous anterior ankle incision, whereas the posterior cysts are approached via a posterolateral incision (**Fig. 5**). The ankle joint and gutters should be debrided, and a synovectomy should be performed where necessary. The metallic components are assessed for stability. If stable, the talus or tibial periprosthetic cyst is approached through a dorsal or anterior window in the adjacent cortex (**Fig. 6**). The cyst is debrided, and the membranous lining is excised (**Fig. 7**). Samples can be sent for histology (hematoxylin and

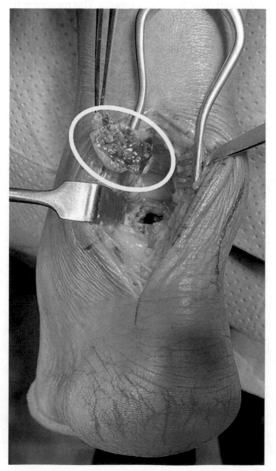

Fig. 7. Membranous lining (demarcated by the *yellow circle*), which was excised from the cyst.

eosin staining, Von Kossa staining, polarized light microscopy, and Oil Red O staining) to try to identify the cause. The walls of the cyst are drilled to allow marrow elements into the cavity. The cyst is then packed with bone graft mixed with DBM (**Fig. 8**). This is done by layering the bone graft and DBM followed by impaction (**Fig. 9**). The authors used to use allograft bone chips but now prefer to use autogenous bone graft when possible. The limited available data suggest better incorporation when using autogenous bone. Intraoperative fluoroscopy is used, to ensure that the cyst is appropriately filled (**Fig. 10**). The metallic components can obscure visualization of the cyst, making it difficult to confirm complete filling of the defect. Lundeen and colleagues[84] recently described the technique of endoscopic-assisted periprosthetic cyst curettage and bone grafting. The scope allows for better visualization of the cysts to confirm adequate debridement and removal of cyst contents and improve bone graft impaction and filling of the void. The PE insert is exchanged whenever possible. The wound is washed out and closed in a routine manner. A below-knee plaster slab is applied. The patients are followed up at 2 weeks for a wound check and placed in a CAM (controlled ankle motion) boot with partial weight-bearing and range-of-motion exercises. The patient is allowed to progress from partial weight-bearing to full weight-bearing as tolerated over the next 4 weeks. The patient is transitioned into conventional shoes at 6 to 8 weeks after surgery.[68]

OUTCOMES OF BONE GRAFTING PERIPROSTHETIC BONE CYSTS

The literature regarding the outcome of periprosthetic cysts bone grafting is limited and inconsistent, especially for asymptomatic cysts. Because of the lack of evidence,

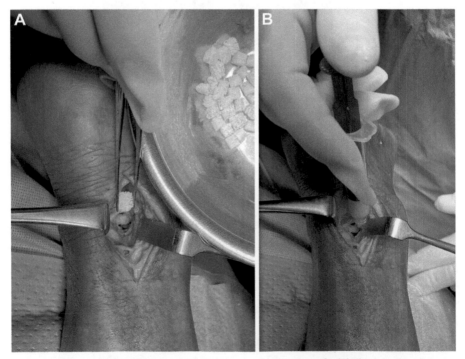

Fig. 8. (*A*) Allograft cancellous bone chips was used as bone graft. (*B*) The bone graft is supplemented with DBM in a layered fashion.

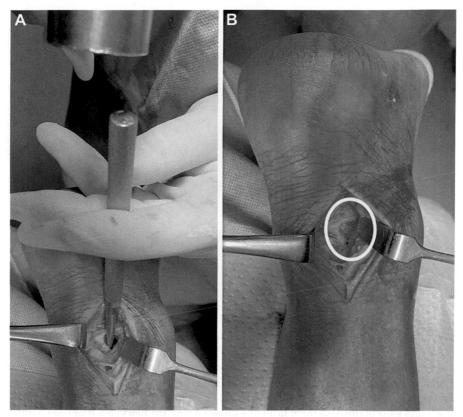

Fig. 9. (*A*) Each layer of bone graft and DBM is impacted using a bone punch. (*B*) The cystic cavity is completely filled with impacted bone graft and DBM (demarcated by the *yellow circle*).

there are no definitive guidelines with regard to size and location for managing asymptomatic periprosthetic cysts surgically. It is important to be careful when analyzing the available literature. The initial large case series were reported on patients with the AES TAA. These studies all reported poor outcomes with bone grafting of periprosthetic bone cysts. Of note, the AES prosthesis was taken off the market in 2008 owing to an abnormally high incidence of periprosthetic osteolysis. The high failure rate with bone grafting in patients with this prosthesis is not necessarily due to the bone grafting procedure but rather to the flaws in the implant itself, which caused a high rate of osteolysis.[16,71]

Mann and colleagues[85] identified 10 patients with periprosthetic cysts in a long-term review of the STAR prosthesis. Four patients had bone grafting of the cysts with no progression or additional radiolucencies seen after a further 5 years of follow-up. Two patients had cysts measuring 5 mm or smaller, which were observed and remained unchanged at 3 years of follow-up. These cysts may have been preoperative degenerative bone cysts, which are thought not to progress. Two patients had cysts of 10 mm in size that enlarged during follow-up. These 2 patients were offered bone grafting but refused additional surgery, as they were asymptomatic. This may be an indicator that periprosthetic cysts of 10 mm or larger have the propensity to enlarge and thus should be managed earlier.

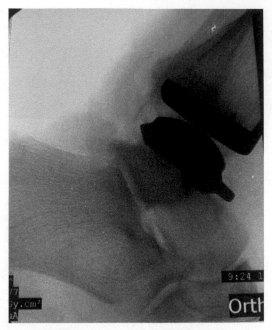

Fig. 10. Fluoroscopy is used to assess for complete grafting of the cyst.

Bonnin and colleagues[12] identified 11 patients with periprosthetic cysts greater than 5 mm in size in their midterm review of 98 Salto Talaris implants. Eight patients had bone grafting of the cysts using autogenous bone from the iliac crest. They reported complete incorporation of bone graft in 4 patients and residual cysts less than 5 mm in size in the remaining 4 patients using radiographs. There was no progression in cyst size or further surgery required.

Yoon and colleagues[24] had a 37.4% (37 patients) incidence of periprosthetic cysts at an average follow-up of 3 years in patients with the Hintegra prosthesis. Ten patients were found to have progression in cyst size during follow-up. Eight patients had bone grafting of the cysts with autogenous bone from the iliac crest. They reported that all osteolytic defects had healed with no signs of progression after 15.3 months of follow-up.

Trincat and colleagues[86] reported on 21 Salto arthroplasties that developed osteolytic lesions, measuring at least 10 mm on one radiographic view, managed with autogenous bone grafting. Six patients had complete resolution of the osteolytic cysts, and 11 patients had significant decrease in cyst size with no progression at 2 years of follow-up. They had a 19% failure rate with 3 patients being converted to an arthrodesis, and one had a revision of the prosthesis.

Yang and colleagues[70] reported a 9% incidence of asymptomatic periprosthetic lytic lesions in a cohort of 210 Hintegra TAAs at a mean follow-up of 6.4 years. These patients were managed with curettage of the cystic lesion, bone grafting, and PE liner exchange. They reported no further progression in these cysts after management. However, they did not mention what type of graft was used or how these patients were followed up.

Gross and colleagues[67] reported 31 (4.3%) patients with periprosthetic cysts larger than 10 mm that were grafted. This cohort included 3 types of prosthesis: STAR, Salto Talaris, and Inbone (Stryker, Kalamazoo, MI). They reported a success rate of 90.9% at 2 years and 60.6% at 4 years. This case series was the largest reporting on the use of allograft, as this was used in 76% of cases. The use of allograft rather than autograft could have contributed to the decrease in success seen at 4 years' follow-up.

Naude and colleagues[68] recently reported the outcome of bone grafting periprosthetic cysts by assessing graft incorporation and cysts progression using CT imaging at 3 years' follow-up. They identified 8 patients with 9 cysts with a volume greater than 1.75 cm^3 (15 mm in all 3 axes) in which 7 patients were bone grafted using allograft bone chips and one with autogenous bone graft from the proximal knee. All bone graft material was supplemented with DBM. They had an 89% mean graft incorporation at 3 years with no reoperation or implant failure and good functional outcomes (**Fig. 11**). Of note, the largest cyst in the cohort was bone grafted with autogenous bone and had 94% graft incorporation, whereas the second largest cyst was grafted with allograft bone chips and only had 69%

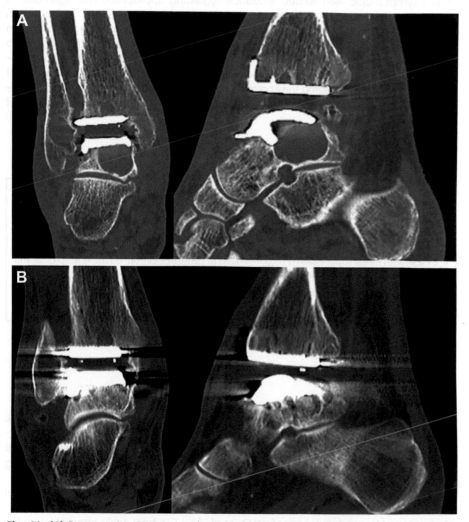

Fig. 11. (A) Preoperative CT scan used to quantify size and location of cyst for operative planning. (B) Follow-up CT scan at 3 years used to assess incorporation of bone graft and cyst progression.

graft incorporation. The authors recommend that autogenous bone graft be used whenever possible.

SUMMARY

TAA has become a popular and viable management option for end-stage ankle arthritis. Improved surgical techniques and implant design are increasing the survivorship of ankle replacements. Aseptic loosening and periprosthetic osteolysis are 2 of the most common causes for reoperation and revision surgery. It is critical to follow up these patients on an annual basis and assess for periprosthetic osteolysis. Routine radiography has been shown to be inferior in detecting these lytic lesions. A CT scan with metal subtraction should be done in all suspected cases to confirm location, quantify lesion size, and aid in surgical planning when indicated. These patients are often asymptomatic with limited evidence regarding appropriate management. In general, smaller lesions should be monitored closely for progression in size, which will then require surgical management. Periprosthetic cysts measuring 10 to 15 mm in all 3 axes should be considered for debridement and curettage with autogenous bone grafting and PE liner exchange. The authors believe that bone grafting of asymptomatic large periprosthetic cysts can be beneficial in preventing implant displacement and failure, thereby increasing the implant survival and functional outcomes.[67,68] Long-term follow-up studies are required to better assess for outcomes in bone grafting of periprosthetic cysts.

CLINICS CARE POINTS

- Periprosthetic cysts are often asymptomatic but a common cause for implant failure in TAA.
- TAA patients should be followed up annually and assessed for possible development of periprosthetic osteolysis.
- Small periprosthetic cysts should be closely monitored for progression in size or causing pain.
- CT scan with metal suppression is recommended to confirm location, quantify lesion size and aid in surgical planning when indicated.
- Periprosthetic cysts measuring 10-15mm in all three axes with stable components should be considered for debridment and curettage with autogenous bone grafting.

DISCLOSURE

The authors have nothing to disclose.

REFERENCES

1. Espinosa N, Klammer G, Wirth SH. Osteolysis in total ankle replacement: how does it work? Foot Ankle Clin 2017;22(2):267–75.
2. Glazebrook M, Daniels T, Younger A, et al. Comparison of health-related quality of life between patients with end-stage ankle and hip arthrosis. J Bone Joint Surg Am 2008;90(3):499–505.
3. Khademi M, Saragas NP, Ferrao PNF. Medium-term results of the HINTEGRA total ankle arthroplasty. J Foot Ankle 2020;14(3):121–8.
4. Lucas y, Hernandez J, Laffenêtre O, et al. AKILE™ total ankle arthroplasty: clinical and CT scan analysis of periprosthetic cysts. Orthop Traumatol Surg Res 2014;100(8):907–15.

5. Brunner S, Barg A, Knupp M, et al. The Scandinavian total ankle replacement: long-term, eleven to fifteen-year, survivorship analysis of the prosthesis in seventy-two consecutive patients. J Bone Joint Surg Am 2013;95:711–8.
6. Glazebrook MA, Arsenault K, Dunbar M. Evidence-based classification of complications in total ankle arthroplasty. Foot Ankle Int 2009;30(10):945–9.
7. Haddad SL, Coetzee JC, Estok R, et al. Intermediate and long-term outcomes of total ankle arthroplasty and ankle arthrodesis. A systematic review of the literature. J Bone Joint Surg Am 2007;89(9):1899–905.
8. Krause FG, Windolf M, Bora B, et al. Impact of complications in total ankle replacement and ankle arthrodesis analyzed with a validated outcome measurement. J Bone Joint Surg Am 2011;93(9):830–9.
9. Zhao H, Yang Y, Yu G, et al. A systematic review of outcome and failure rate of uncemented Scandinavian Total Ankle Replacement. Int Orthop 2011;35(12):1751–8.
10. Kohonen I, Koivu H, Pudas T, et al. Does computed tomography add information on radiographic analysis in detecting periprosthetic osteolysis after total ankle arthroplasty? Foot Ankle Int 2013;24(2):180–8.
11. Besse JL, Brito N, Lienhart C. Clinical evaluation and radiographic assessment of bone lysis of the AES total ankle replacement. Foot Ankle Int 2009;30(10):964–75.
12. Bonnin M, Gaudot F, Laurent JR, et al. The Salto total ankle arthroplasty: survivorship and analysis of failures at 7 to 11 years. Clin Orthop Relat Res 2011;469:225–36.
13. Deleu PA, Devos Bevernage B, Gombault V, et al. Intermediate-term results of mobile-bearing total ankle replacement. Foot Ankle Int 2015;36(5):518–30.
14. Hanna RS, Haddad SL, Lazarus ML. Evaluation of periprosthetic lucency after total ankle arthroplasty: helical CT versus conventional radiography. Foot Ankle Int 2007;28(8):921–6.
15. Jensen J, Frøkjær J, Gerke O, et al. Evaluation of periprosthetic bone cysts in patients with a Scandinavian total ankle replacement: weight-bearing conventional digital radiographs versus weight-bearing multiplanar reconstructed fluoroscopic imaging. AJR Am J Roentgenol 2014;203(4):863–8.
16. Kohonen IA, Koivu H, Tiusanen H, et al. Are periprosthetic osteolytic lesions in ankle worth bone grafting? Foot Ankle Surg 2017;23:128–33.
17. Koivu H, Kohonen IA, Mattila K, et al. Medium to long term results of 130 Ankle Evolutive System total ankle replacements – inferior survival due to peri-implant osteolysis. Foot Ankle Surg 2017;23:108–15.
18. Koivu H, Kohonen I, Sipola E, et al. Severe periprosthetic osteolytic lesions after the Ankle Evolutive System total ankle replacement. J Bone Joint Surg Br 2009;91:907–14.
19. Kokkonen A, Ikävalko M, Tiihonen R, et al. High rate of osteolytic lesions in medium-term followup after the AES total ankle replacement. Foot Ankle Int 2011;32(2):168–75.
20. Kopp FJ, Patel MM, Deland JT, et al. Total ankle arthroplasty with the Agility prosthesis: clinical and radiographic evaluation. Foot Ankle Int 2006;27(2):97–103.
21. Lintz F, Mast J, Bernasconi A, Mehdi N, de Cesar Netto C, Fernando C, Buedts K, International Weight Bearing CT Society. 3D, weightbearing topographical study of periprosthetic cysts and alignment in total ankle replacement. Foot Ankle Int 2020;4(1):1–9.
22. Mulcahy H, Chew FS. Current concepts in total ankle replacements for radiologists: complications. AJR Am J Roentgenol 2015;205(6):1244–50.

23. Schutte BG, Louwerens JW. Short-term results of our first 49 Scandinavian total ankle replacements (STAR). Foot Ankle Int 2008;29(2):124–7.
24. Yoon HS, Lee J, Choi WJ, et al. Periprosthetic osteolysis after total ankle arthroplasty. Foot Ankle Int 2014;35(1):14–21.
25. Day J, Kim J, O'Mally MJ, et al. Radiographic and clinical outcomes of the Salto Talaris Total ankle arthroplasty. Foot Ankle Int 2020;41(12):1519–28.
26. Arcangelo J, Guerra-Pinto F, Pinto A, et al. Peri-prosthetic bone cysts after total ankle replacement. A systematic review and meta-analysis. Foot Ankle Surg 2019;25:96–105.
27. Lavernia CJ. Cost-effectiveness of early surgical intervention in silent osteolysis. J Arthroplasty 1998;13(3):277–9.
28. Schenk K, Lieske S, John M, et al. Prospective study of a cementless, mobile-bearing, third generation total ankle prosthesis. Foot Ankle Int 2011;32(8):755–63.
29. Najefi A, Ghani Y, Goldberg A. Bone cysts and osteolysis in ankle replacement. Foot Ankle Int 2021;42(1):55–61.
30. Chiba K, Burghardt AJ, Osaki M, et al. Three-dimensional analysis of subchondral cysts in hip osteoarthritis: an ex vivo HR-pQCT study. Bone 2014;66:140–5.
31. Freund E. The pathological significance of intra-articular pressure. Edinburgh Med J 1940;47:192.
32. Resnick D, Niwayama G, Coutts RD. Subchondral cysts (geodes) in arthritic disorders: pathologic and radiographic appearance of the hip joint. AJR Am J Roentgenol 1977;128(5):799–806.
33. RHANEY K, LAMB DW. The cysts of osteoarthritis of the hip; a radiological and pathological study. J Bone Joint Surg Br 1955 Nov 1;37-B(4):663–75.
34. Crema MD, Roemer FW, Zhu Y, et al. Subchondral cyst like lesions develop longitudinally in areas of bone marrow edema-like lesions in patients with or at risk for knee osteoarthritis: detection with MR imaging—the MOST study. Radiology 2010 Sep 1;256(3):855–62.
35. Hsu AR, Haddad SL, Myerson MS. Evaluation and management of the painful total ankle arthroplasty. J Am Acad Orthop Surg 2015;23(5):272–82.
36. Dalat F, Barnoud R, Fessy M, et al, French Association of Foot Surgery AFCP. Histologic study of periprosthetic osteolytic lesions after AES total ankle replacement. A 22 case series. Orthop Traumatol Res 2013;99:S285–95.
37. Barg A, Knupp M, Henninger HB, et al. Total ankle replacement using HINTEGRA, an unconstrained, three-component system. Surgical technique and pitfalls. Foot Ankle Clin N Am 2012;17:607–35.
38. Barg A, Zwicky L, Knupp M, et al. Hintegra total ankle replacement: survivorship analysis in 684 patients. J Bone Joint Surg 2013;95(13):1175–83.
39. Huang C-H, Liau J-J, Cheng C-K. Fixed or mobile-bearing total knee arthroplasty. J Orthop Surg Res 2007;2:1.
40. Huang CH, Ho FY, Ma HM, et al. Particle size and morphology of UHMWPE wear debris in failed total knee arthroplasties – a comparison between mobile bearing and fixed bearing knees. J Orthop Res 2002;20:1038–41.
41. Huang C-H, Huang C-H, Liau J-J, et al. Specific complications of the mobile-bearing total knee prosthesis. J Long Term Eff Med Implants 2009;19:1–11.
42. Lu Y-C, Huang C-H, Chang T-K, et al. Wear-pattern analysis in retrieved tibial inserts of mobile-bearing and fixed-bearing total knee prostheses. J Bone Jt Surg Br 2010;92:500–7.
43. Cottrino S, Fabrègue D, Cowie AP, et al. Wear study of total ankle replacement explants by microstructural analysis. J Mech Behav Biomed Mater 2016;61:1–11.

44. Singh G, Reichard T, Hameister R, et al. Ballooning osteolysis in 71 failed total ankle arthroplasties. Acta Orthop 2016;87(4):401–5.
45. Fahlgren A, Bostrom MP, Yang X, et al. Fluid pressure and flow as a cause of bone resorption. Acta Orthop 2010;81:508–16.
46. Rodriguez D, Bevernage BD, Maldague P, et al. Medium term follow-up of the AES ankle prosthesis: high rate of asymptomatic osteolysis. Foot Ankle Surg 2010;16:54–60.
47. Schmalzried TP, Jasty M, Harris WH. Periprosthetic bone loss in total hip arthroplasty. Polyethylene wear debris and the concept of the effective joint space. J Bone Joint Surg Am 1992;74:849–63.
48. Claus AM, Engh CA Jr, Sychterz CJ, et al. Radiographic definition of pelvic osteolysis following total hip arthroplasty. J Bone Joint Surg Am 2003;85(8):1519–26.
49. Espinosa N, Walti M, Favre P, et al. Misalignment of total ankle components can induce high joint contact pressures. J Bone Joint Surg Am 2010;92(5):1179–87.
50. Lefrancois T, Younger A, Wing K, et al. A prospective study of four total ankle arthroplasty implants by non-designer investigators. J Bone Joint Surg Am 2017;99(4):342–8.
51. Easley ME, Vertullo CJ, Urban WC, et al. Total ankle arthroplasty. J Am Acad Orthop Surg 2002;10(3):157–67.
52. Nunley JA, Adams SB, Easley ME, et al. Prospective randomized trial comparing mobile-bearing and fixed-bearing total ankle replacement. Foot Ankle Int 2019;40(11):1239–48.
53. Fukuda T, Haddad SL, Ren Y, et al. Impact of talar component rotation on contact pressure after total ankle arthroplasty: a cadaveric study. Foot Ankle Int 2010;31(5):404–11.
54. Rush SM, Todd N. Salto Talaris fixed-bearing total ankle replacement system. Clin Podiatr Med Surg 2013;30:69–80.
55. Schipper ON, Haddad SL, Pytel P, et al. Histological analysis of early osteolysis in total ankle arthroplasty. Foot Ankle Int 2017;38(4):351–9.
56. van Wijngaarden R, van der Plaat L, Nieuwe Weme RA, et al. Etiopathogenesis of osteolytic cysts associated with total ankle arthroplasty, a histological study. Foot Ankle Surg 2015;21(2):132–6.
57. Gaden MT, Ollivere BJ. Periprosthetic aseptic osteolysis in total ankle replacement: cause and management. Clin Podiatr Med Surg 2013;30(2):145–55.
58. Mehta N, Serino J, Hur ES, et al. Pathogenesis, evaluation and management of osteolysis following total ankle arthroplasty. Foot Ankle Int 2021;42(2):230–42.
59. Matthews JB, Green TR, Stone MH, et al. Comparison of the response of three human monocytic cell lines to challenge with polyethylene particles of known size and dose. J Mater Sci Mater Med 2001;12(3):249–58.
60. Goodman SB. The effects of micromotion and particulate materials on tissue differentiation. Bone chamber studies in rabbits. Acta Orthop Scand Suppl 1994;258:1–43.
61. Kienapfel H, Sprey C, Wilke A, et al. Implant fixation by bone ingrowth. J Arthroplasty 1999;14(3):355–68.
62. McInnes KA, Younger AS, Oxland TR. Initial instability in total ankle replacement: a cadaveric biomechanical investigation of the STAR and agility prostheses. J Bone Joint Surg Am 2014;96(17):e147.
63. Knecht SI, Estin M, Callaghan JJ, et al. The agility total ankle arthroplasty. Seven to sixteen-year follow-up. J Bone Joint Surg 2004;86-A:1161–71.

64. Gruen TA, Mcneice GM, Amstutz HC. "Modes of failure" of cemented stem type femoral components: a radiographic analysis of loosening. Clin Orthop Relat Res 1979;141:17–27.

65. Bischoff JE, Fryman JC, Parcell J, et al. Influence of crosslinking on the wear performance of polyethylene within total ankle arthroplasty. Foot Ankle Int 2015; 36(4):369–76.

66. Hernandez JL, Laffenetre O, Toullec E, et al. AKILE total ankle arthroplasty: Clinical and CT scan analysis of periprosthetic cysts. Orthop Traumatol Surg Res 2014;100:907–15.

67. Gross CE, Huh J, Green C, et al. Outcomes of bone grafting of bone cysts after total ankle arthroplasty. Foot Ankle Int 2016;37(2):157–64.

68. Naude JJ, Saragas NP, Ferrao PN. CT scan assessment and functional outcome of periprosthetic bone grafting after total ankle arthroplasty at medium-term follow-up. Foot Ankle Int 2022;43(5):609–19.

69. Bai LB, Lee KB, Song EK, et al. Total ankle arthroplasty outcome comparison for post-traumatic and primary osteoarthritis. Foot Ankle Int 2010;31(12):1048–56.

70. Yang HY, Wang SH, Lee KB. The HINTEGRA total ankle arthroplasty: functional outcomes and implant survivorship in 210 osteoarthritic ankles at a mean of 6.4 years. Bone Joint Lett J 2019;101-B:695–701.

71. Besse JL, Lienhart C, Fessy M. Outcomes following cyst curettage and bone grafting for the management of periprosthetic cyst evolution after AES total ankle replacement. Clin Podiatr Med Surg 2013;30:157–70.

72. Kim DR, Choi YS, Potter HG, et al. Total ankle arthroplasty: an imaging overview. Korean J Radiol 2016;17(3):413–23.

73. Hintermann B, Zwicky L, Knupp M, et al. HINTEGRA revision arthroplasty for failed total ankle prostheses. J Bone Joint Surg Am 2013;95(13):1166–74.

74. Fuchs S, Sandmann C, Skwara A, et al. Quality of life 20 years after arthrodesis of the ankle. A study of adjacent joints. J Bone Joint Surg Br 2003;85(7):994–8.

75. Jeng CL, Campbell JT, Tang EY, et al. Tibiotalocalcaneal arthrodesis with bulk femoral head allograft for salvage of large defects in the ankle. Foot Ankle Int 2013;34(9):1256–66.

76. Coetzee JC, Den Hartog BD, McGaver RS, et al. Femoral head allografts for talar body defects. Foot Ankle Int 2021;42(7):1–9.

77. Abar B, Kwon N, Allen NB, et al. Outcomes of Surgical Reconstruction Using Custom 3D-Printed Porous Titanium Implants for Critical-Sized Bone Defects of the Foot and Ankle. Foot Ankle Int 2022;43(6). https://doi.org/10.1177/10711007 221077113.

78. Carlsson AS, Montgomery F, Besjakov J. Arthrodesis of the ankle secondary to replacement. Foot Ankle Int 1998;19(4):240–5.

79. Hopgood P, Kumar R, Wood PL. Ankle arthrodesis for failed total ankle replacement. J Bone Joint Surg Br 2006;88(8):1032–8.

80. Jehan S, Hill SO. Operative technique of two parallel compression screws and autologous bone graft for ankle arthrodesis after failed total ankle replacement. Foot Ankle Int 2012;33(9):767–71.

81. Kitaoka HB, Romness DW. Arthrodesis for failed ankle arthroplasty. J Arthroplasty 1992;7(3):277–84.

82. Henry JK, Rider C, Cody E, et al. Evaluating and managing the painful Total ankle replacement. Foot and ankle international 2021. https://doi.org/10.1177/107110 07211027273.

83. Rodrigues-Pinto R, Muras J, Martín Oliva X, et al. Functional results and complication analysis after total ankle replacement. Early to medium-term results from a

Portuguese and Spanish prospective multicentric study. Foot Ankle Surg 2013; 19:222–8.

84. Lundeen GA, Barousse PS, Moles LH, et al. Technique Tip: Endoscopic assisted curettage and bon grafting of periprosthetic total ankle arthroplasty bone cysts. Foot Ankle Int 2021;42(2):224–9.

85. Mann Jeffrey A, Mann Roger A, Horton Eric. STAR™ Ankle: Long-Term Results. Foot Ankle Int 2011;32(5):473–84.

86. Trincat S, Gaudot F, Lavigne F, et al. Total ankle prostheses and geodes: results of autologous bone transplants at more than 2 years. Rev Chir Orthop Traumatol 2011;97:S328–9.

Diagnosing and Managing Infection in Total Ankle Replacement

Markus Walther, MD[a,b,c,d,*], Veit Krenn, MD[e], Kathrin Pfahl, MD[a,b]

KEYWORDS

- Infection • Total ankle replacement • Revision

KEY POINTS

- Periprosthetic joint infection after total ankle replacement (TAR) can be classified into acute and chronic infections.
- Proof of difficult-to-treat (DTT) bacteria with resistance against biofilm-active antibiotics leads to a 2-stage revision procedure with the removal of the hardware.
- Early infections with not-DTT bacteria (<4 weeks after implantation) can be managed successfully with 1 or several debridements, irrigation, and a change of polyethylene inlay.
- Late and chronic infections require implant removal.
- Chronic pain and early loosening after TAR are likely signs of a low-grade infection, even with normal inflammatory blood parameters and negative findings in aspirated joint fluid.
- Intraoperative diagnostics should include at least 5 samples for microbiology and 5 samples for histology with additional sonication of the removed implant (2 samples from the tibia interface, 2 samples from the talar interface, 1 sample from the capsule).
- Antibiotics can only support but not replace surgical treatment. Biofilm-active antibiotics are needed in patients treated with irrigation, debridement, and polyethylene exchange but implant retention. Moreover, biofilm-active antibiotics should be considered after the definitive surgical treatment.

[a] Department of Foot and Ankle Surgery, Schön Klinik München Harlaching — FIFA Medical Centre, Harlachinger Straße 51, Munich 81547, Germany; [b] Department of Orthopaedics and Trauma Surgery, Musculoskeletal University Center Munich (MUM), University Hospital, LMU Munich, Marchioninistraße 15, München 81377, Germany; [c] Department of Orthopedic Surgery, University of Wuerzburg, Brettreichstrasse 11, Würzburg 97074, Germany; [d] Paracelsus Medical University, Strubergasse 21, Salzburg 5020, Austria; [e] Pathologie Trier, Max-Planck-Str. 5, Trier 54296, Germany
* Corresponding author. Center for Foot and Ankle Surgery, Schön Klinik München Harlaching, Harlachinger Straße 51, Munich 81547, Germany.
E-mail address: mwalther@schoen-klinik.de

Foot Ankle Clin N Am 29 (2024) 145–156
https://doi.org/10.1016/j.fcl.2023.09.002
1083-7515/24/

BACKGROUND AND DEFINITIONS

The frequency of infection after total ankle arthroplasty (TAR) reported in the literature is between 0.5% and 8.9%.[1-7] A recently published article by Sambandam and colleagues[8] analyzed the differences in complication rates between TAR and ankle arthrodesis (AA). They found a significantly higher infection rate after AA (5.9%) than TAR (4.1%) after the first postoperative year. The results are remarkable because of the vast cohort in the 2 matched groups, including 657 females and 630 males. Different indications for TAR and AA can explain the higher infection rate for AA. Similar findings have been reported in a meta-analysis by Almutairo and colleagues.[9]

The following risk factors may predispose a patient to an infection after TAR and should alert the surgeon in the case of failure. Risk factors include inflammatory arthritis,[10,11] prior ankle surgery,[5] body mass index (BMI) less than 19, and peripheral vascular disease.[11] Other possible risk factors discussed in the literature are obesity (BMI>30),[11] tobacco use,[11-13] diabetes,[11,13-15] duration of surgery,[5,13] age less than 65 years,[11] hypothyroidism, low preoperative American Orthopaedic Foot & Ankle Society Hindfoot Score,[5] and chronic lung disease.[11,16]

Zhang and colleagues[17] tested the usability of the Mayo Periprosthetic Joint Infection Risk Score for TAR. They found that the Mayo Score could predict the risk for PJI after TAA as precisely as after total hip and knee arthroplasty.

Periprosthetic joint infection (PJI) can be classified into 3 categories[18]: acute PJI (which can be divided into early perioperative with onset earlier than 4 weeks after surgery and acute hematogenous with <4 weeks of symptoms) and chronic PJI with onset 4 or more weeks after surgery or duration of symptoms of 4 or more weeks.

Since biofilm formation plays an essential role in the pathogenesis of PJI, bacteria resistant to biofilm-active antibiotics (eg, rifampicin) are classified as difficult to treat (DTT).[19]

Staphylococcus species are the most common cultured microorganisms in recent studies, and the reported microbiological findings were consistent with PJI in the hip and knee.[20]

In 2017, we published a paper on the histologic classification of TAR failure in analogy to the methods used for endoprosthesis failure in the knee and hip.[21,22] The research underscored the importance of histologic examination as an essential tool in implant revision surgery. Synovia-like interface membrane (SLIM) type II or III represents TAR failure caused by infection (**Table 1**).

Many articles on the revision of TAR report a significant rate of patients with "pain without another cause." In their revision TAR (R-TAR) study, Richter and colleagues[25] found 12% within this category. However, this category is based on clinical findings and sometimes microbiologic analysis. Detailed histologic results are not reported in most of the papers. After starting a detailed microbiologic and histologic analysis of the periprosthetic tissue, those unclear cases decreased dramatically. Meanwhile, we are convinced that low-grade infection in TAR is significantly underreported, and many cases with unclear pain are just unrecognized low-grade infections.

PRESURGICAL DIAGNOSTICS

Patients suspicious of PJI are characterized by clinical features such as pain, swelling, inflammation, or persistent wound problems. More obvious clinical signs include the presence of a sinus tract (fistula) or purulence around the prosthesis. There can be elevated infectious parameters in the laboratory. If radiograph show cysts, lysis, signs of loosening, or ossifications, the suspicion of infection is further substantiated.

Table 1
Histopathological diagnosis and classification of total ankle replacement failure[21–24]

SLIM		Histologic Findings	Clinical Findings
SLIM type I	Particle type	Confluent infiltrate of macrophages (often with foamy features) and multinuclear giant cells. Prosthesis wear. Particles>5 μm found in multinuclear giant cells, particles<1 μm in macrophages and extracellular localization.	Cystic lesions.
SLIM type II	Infectious type	Low-grade: granulation tissue with fibroblasts, reactive vascular proliferation, chronic edema, and an inflammatory infiltrate made of neutrophil granulocytes, plasma cells as well as small lymphocytic aggregates. CD15 focus score>39 cells per HPF. High-grade: high number of neutrophil granulocytes. CD15 focus score >106 cells per HPF	TAR failure with septic loosening (high grade and low grade).
SLIM type III	Combined type	Combination of particle-induced and infectious neo-synovium/ periprosthetic membrane (types I and II). Wear particle–induced reaction as well as of bacterial infection in the same tissue. CD15 focus score>39 cells per HPF	Cystic lesions with features of infection.
SLIM type IV	Indifferent type	No evidence of wear particles or inflammatory infiltrates indicating a bacterial infection. Connective tissue with high collagen content, surface layer like the synovial lining. Abrasion particles are non-detectable or are present only in small quantity. CD15 focus score <39 cells per HPF	Loosening of TAR without cysts or histologic features of infection.
SLIM type V	Arthrofibrosis, particle-induced and not particle-induced	Fibroblast reaction and fibrosis with a high fibroblast cellularity and>20 β-catenin-positive fibroblasts per HPF. CD15 focus score <39 cells per HPF	Stiff joint with significant fibrotic tissue.
SLIM type VI	Inflammatory inverse reactions	Toxic or allergic reaction to the implant material. Severe lymphocyte/macrophage infiltration, necrosis, abrasion particle detection, and granuloma formation.	Adverse and allergic reaction
SLIM type VII	Bone pathologies	Local osteopenia, aseptic bone necrosis, inflammatory reactions due to intramedullary particle reactions and ossification.	Loosening or pain caused by heterotopic ossification or periarticular osteopenia.

Abbreviations: CD15 focus score CD, cluster of differentiation; EAF, endoprosthesis-associated arthrofibrosis; HPF, high-power field; SLIM, Synovia-like interface membrane; TAR, total ankle replacement.

These findings should lead to synovial fluid aspiration to determine the leukocyte count and the percentage of granulocytes and to inoculate a microbiological culture.[26] Problematic at the ankle joint is the small volume of synovial fluid. Sometimes it is not possible to aspirate any fluid. In this case, it is possible to inject some saline and aspirate the saline for microbiology. In our approach, we have switched to pediatric blood cultures to decrease the amount of fluid needed and increase the detection rate of microbiological samples. If we have enough joint aspirate, we use urine test strips to check for leukocyte esterase, another indicator of PJI.[27,28]

Imaging techniques such as PET-computed tomography or metal suppression MRI are helpful when various differential diagnoses are considered.[29]

If the analyses confirm any infection, revision of the prosthesis is indicated. If the results are inconsistent, for example, if the aspirate is negative, but a high clinical suspicion is still present, taking periprosthetic probes with or without removing components or the complete implant should be considered.

Any antibiotic treatment should be avoided until the intraoperative samples are taken. The uncontrolled use of antibiotics prior to adequate diagnostics often compromises microbiological investigation and limits the validity of the laboratory results.

INTRAOPERATIVE DIAGNOSTICS

Intraoperatively, at least 5 samples should be taken for microbiological and histologic analyses. Two samples should be from the tibial, 2 from the talar interface, and 1 from the capsule. If possible, antibiotics should not have been administered prior to sampling. A blood culture bottle can also be used for intraoperative sampled synovial fluid. As soon as any prosthesis component is removed, including the polyethylene inlay, it should be sent for sonication for further analysis.[30] Multiplex polymerase chain reaction of sonication fluid is a good test for diagnosing PJI, particularly in patients who previously received antibiotics, and further helps to get a precise diagnosis.[31,32] Microbiological samples should be inoculated for at least 14 days.

Barrack and colleagues[33] reported on unexpected positive intraoperative cultures in a series of revision total knee replacements. They found 41 cases with positive cultures out of 692 total cases. Based on their finding, the authors recommended sending at least 5 sets of cultures in the setting of abnormal preoperative inflammatory markers, abnormal synovial aspirate, or tissue appearing concerning for infection intraoperatively at the time of revision.

The article of Jacobs and colleagues[34] inspired us to start a more thorough search for low-grade infections. They reported 679 cases of revision hip or knee arthroplasty for presumed aseptic failure with an incidence of unsuspected infection of 10% detected by samples taken intraoperatively.

As part of a consensus statement of the 2018 International Consensus Meeting of Musculoskeletal Infection, Fuchs recommends intraoperative cultures as a routine procedure during revision total ankle arthroplasty.[35]

Because microbiology can be negative for several reasons, including the uncontrolled use of antibiotics by the patient, we always take histologic samples. We grade the periprosthetic membrane according to the classification system published by Krenn and Morawietz.[22] CD15-score, as a more recent histologic method, can be determined in more ambiguous cases.[23]

TYPICAL BACTERIA IN TOTAL ANKLE REPLACEMENT INFECTION

There is a paucity of literature on bacteria found in TAR infection. We analyzed and published our cases in 2022.[36] The most common pathogen in our cases of acute infection was *Staphylococcus aureus* (67%), followed by *S caprae* (16%). 17% were polymicrobial.

We found 77% coagulase-negative staphylococci and 8% *Bacillus* species in chronic and low-grade infection. 15% of the chronic cases were polymicrobial.[36]

SURGICAL MANAGEMENT OF TOTAL ANKLE REPLACEMENT INFECTION
Irrigation and Debridement

Implant-preserving treatment options include irrigation and debridement (I&D) alone and I&D with polyethylene exchange. The indication to try an implant-preserving strategy is the acute infection with bacteria sensitive to biofilm-active antibiotics and no signs of implant loosening.[36]

In our hands, it is technically nearly impossible to perform I&D of all regions of the ankle joint without removing the polyethylene inlay. Therefore, preservation of the inlay does not play a role in our treatment concept. Although the failure rate of I&D with polyethylene exchange is significantly higher than after the removal of all implants, it is less invasive, and successful infection management is possible.[37] In addition, an I&D procedure is an excellent opportunity to take further probes for microbiology and histology from the joint capsule and to send the removed polyethylene inlay for sonication in unclear cases.

One-Stage Revision

We consider a 1-stage revision to ankle fusion in chronic infections with not-DTT bacteria. When the patient urges us toward R-TAR, we feel more comfortable with a 2-stage approach, even in not-DTT bacteria.

Two-Stage Revision

Any infection with DTT bacteria is treated with a complete 2-stage revision procedure. Unclear cases with a suspected infection but without final proof prior to surgery are also more suitable for 2-stage revisions. This includes patients with early TAR loosening and pain of unclear cause after TAR.

We take at least 5 samples for microbiological and histologic analyses (2 samples from the tibial interface, 2 from the talar interface, and 1 from the capsule). Synovial fluid is collected in a blood culture bottle for further microbiological investigation. All removed implant components are sent for sonication.[30] Especially in those cases, we have found a high rate of low-grade infections after a careful workup.

When a low-grade infection is suspected clinically, but we do not know the specimen at the time of revision surgery, we use a gentamicin-vancomycin–loaded antibiotic spacer as it covers most of the viable bacteria. If it turns out that we have chosen the wrong antibiotic loading, a change of the bone cement spacer can be mandatory, resulting in 3-stage exchange.

Amputation or definitive treatment with cement spacers should be discussed if those concepts fail.

Intraoperative Antibiotics

Any antibiotic treatment should be avoided until the intraoperative samples are taken. The uncontrolled use of antibiotics prior to adequate diagnostics often compromises microbiological investigation and limits the validity of the laboratory results. We administer perioperative antibiotics according to susceptibility after having taken all the samples. The empiric treatment is ampicillin/sulbactam. If patients present septic or with a positive methicillin-resistant *S aureus* status, history of multiple surgeries, or suspected low-grade infection, ampicillin/sulbactam is combined with vancomycin.

Final Treatment with Revision Total Ankle Replacement or Fusion

In most cases, we remove the bone cement spacer and perform fusion or R-TAR after 6 weeks. At this point, all clinical signs of infections should have settled. A second period with an antibiotic-loaded bone cement spacer can be mandatory for persistent clinical signs of infection.

As functional differences are minor in patient-reported outcome measures, we feel more comfortable performing an ankle fusion after infection than performing R-TAR.[38] However, an increasing number of patients request R-TAR, especially if they have had a good experience with their implant before. At this stage, there is no evidence for a recommendation. In our hands, R-TAR is a viable option as long as bone stock and the soft tissues are suitable.

To eradicate any persistent bacteria and to protect the newly implanted metal after revision surgery, biofilm-active antibiotics are administered intravenously for 1 week and another 5 weeks orally.

ANTIBIOTICS

The major challenge of PJI is the biofilm on the implant.[39] Therefore, biofilm-active therapy is mandatory, especially in implant-preserving strategies like I&D with polyethylene exchange and after R-TAR or fusion. A biofilm-active therapy for staphylococci infection consists of rifampicin, supplemented with a second antibiotic to prevent resistance formation. Fluoroquinolones with proper gram-positive action work well in this indication (ie, levofloxacin, moxifloxacin); however, other antibiotics with good bioavailability and bone penetration may be as adequate.[40]

Although rifampicin showed promising activity in in vitro biofilms, antibiotics can only support the surgical strategy, which is the most important predictor for clinical outcomes. There is some evidence from PJI of the knee that the optimal start of rifampicin administration is between days 5 and 9 after surgery.[41]

Fluoroquinolones have good activity against biofilms produced by gram-negative bacteria. These in vitro findings are supported by clinical studies demonstrating the effect of fluoroquinolones as a first-line antibiotic treatment for PJIs caused by gram-negative bacteria.

Antibiotic treatment duration should be 3 months for acute PJIs treated with I&D with implant retention. In revision surgery with implant removal and a hardware-free period of 6 weeks, another 6 weeks of antibiotic treatment after the definitive surgical treatment is probably sufficient.[40,42]

Intravenous antibiotics can be switched to an oral treatment regimen after 2 weeks, provided an antibiotic with anti-biofilm properties and adequate bioavailability is available.[43]

After implant removal with a gentamicin-vancomycin–loaded cement spacer implantation, antibiotics are chosen in cooperation with the infectious disease specialist according to the microbiological findings. Antibiotic therapy is generally more straightforward after implant removal as a high level of gentamicin and vancomycin is locally delivered by the spacer. Moreover, removing the implant solves the problem of biofilm and enlarges the range of possible antibiotics. Long-term suppression therapies for more than 12 months are known treatment concepts in PJI after total knee or hip replacement. In PJI of TAR, we consider fusion a better option than long-term antibiotics.

For an even more detailed discussion of different antibiotic concepts, we refer to the pocket guide "Periprosthetic joint infections," issued by the Pro-Implant Foundation, a European non-profit nongovernmental organization dealing with all kinds of implant-associated infections in medicine.[44]

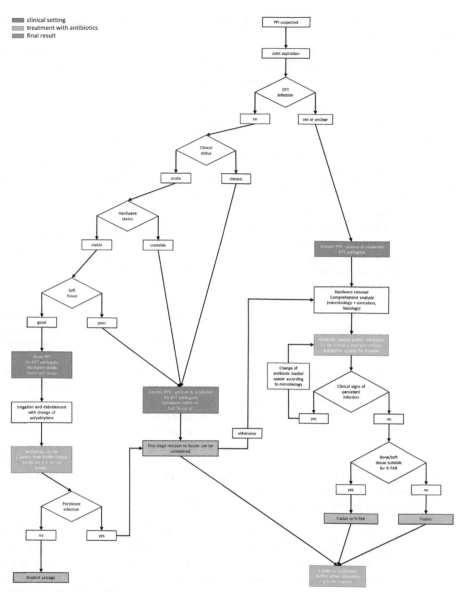

Fig. 1. Preferred treatment algorithm. DDT, difficult to treat infection caused by pathogens resistant to biofilm active antibiotics; i.v., administered intravenous; p.o., administered oral; PPJ, periprosthetic joint infection.

DISCUSSION

In acute PJI, high-virulent bacteria such as *S aureus* are primarily responsible for the infection. Chronic PJIs are typically associated with low-virulent bacteria such as coagulase-negative staphylococci.[18] With new diagnostic procedures like implant sonication and prolonged culture incubation, a higher detection rate of low-virulent bacteria such as *Cutibacterium* spp. can be expected in the future.[45]

These new data might lead to a shift in the spectrum of pathogens requiring a different approach.

In chronic PJI after total hip and knee arthroplasty, there is still a debate on whether 1-stage or 2-stage revisions have better results. In a recently published systematic review and meta-analysis by Goud and colleagues,[46] the reinfection rates following 1-stage and 2-stage hip and knee arthroplasty revisions were similar.

For the ankle, there are no data available. D'Errico and colleagues[47] concluded that it is impossible to give any recommendations based on the few low-quality articles on this topic. In their analysis, the overlapping of confidence intervals related to all analyzed interventions showed no superiority of either technique.

However, there is some evidence that implant removal produces more reliable results than I&D. Kessler and colleagues described a 100% rate of infection-free survival in 9 patients treated with a 2-stage revision procedure, while 21 PJIs with retention of 1 or both components resulted in a 66.7% rate of infection-free survival.[48]

We found a 40% failure rate in cases with acute infections treated with I&D and polyethylene exchange.[36] Another study showed similar results with a 54% long-term failure rate after a mean follow-up of 2.8 ± 1.5 years in 14 patients with acute hematogenous PJI who underwent I&D and polyethylene exchange.[37] Patton and colleagues treated acute infections successfully with polyethylene exchange in 2 cases and debridement alone in 3 cases.[13]

Myerson and colleagues reported on 4 acute infections of TAA treated with I&D and polyethylene exchange. All 4 cases suffered from recurrent infection.[6] Although these cohorts are small, they demonstrate the limitations of I&D with or without polyethylene exchange.

The next question is whether the definitive treatment should be ankle fusion or if it might be an indication for R-TAR when the infection has settled. Myerson and colleagues examined 7 patients who received a revision arthroplasty, and the procedure was successful in only 3 patients resulting in a success rate of 16%, whereas all 6 patients who converted to arthrodesis showed successful results.[6]

Making an evidence-based recommendation regarding ankle fusion and R-TAR is still impossible. Based on our experience, we feel more comfortable recommending arthrodesis than performing R-TAR after PJI, especially considering the minor functional differences between the 2 options.[38]

If AA is the preferred solution after PJI after TAR, the final question arises whether these cases might have experienced a more favorable outcome if they had been converted to an ankle fusion right away rather than performing a 2-stage revision. Stage revision surgeries are invasive, with a prolonged postoperative course and an inevitable loss of bone stock, limiting future treatment options. At this stage, there is no evidence in either direction. We have to carefully discuss the different options, chances, and limitations of the different treatment options with the patient to find an individual solution for the challenging problem of PJI. Our preferred treatment algorithm is shown in **Fig. 1**, although not all decisions are evidence based.

SUMMARY

Infections after TAR are one of the most challenging situations for the treating physician. Early infections within the first 4 weeks after implantation can be managed successfully with 1 or several debridements, irrigation, and a change of polyethylene inlay in combination with biofilm-active antibiotics. Chronic infections require implant removal. A careful assessment is mandatory to identify low-grade infections, which can be missed in the preoperative laboratory and joint aspiration. Especially early aseptic loosening and ankle pain without an apparent reason are suspicious for low-grade infection.

Several surgical concepts are possible, including 1-stage revisions and 2-stage revisions using an antibiotic spacer. After the infection has settled, the final treatment is either revision arthroplasty or ankle fusion. Although single-surgery revisions are reported in the literature, our experience with 2-stage revisions using an antibiotics-loaded bone cement spacer is better. This concept allows comprehensive microbiologic and histologic investigations. Besides the results of those investigations, bone stock and soft tissue conditions are the most critical factor for the final decision between fusion and R-TAR.

CLINICS CARE POINTS

- PJI after TAR can be classified into acute and chronic infections.
- Early infections (<4 weeks after implantation) can be managed successfully with 1 or several debridements, irrigation, and a change of polyethylene inlay.
- Late and chronic infections require implant removal. The major challenge in those infections is biofilm-producing bacteria.
- Bacteria resistant to biofilm-active antibiotics are DTT specimens. DTT infections require complete implant removal and the implantation of an antibiotic-loaded spacer.
- A low-grade infection must be considered in patients with chronic pain or early loosening after TAR, even with normal inflammatory blood parameters and negative findings in aspirated joint fluid.
- Intraoperative diagnostics should include at least 5 samples for microbiology and 5 samples for histology with additional sonication of the removed implant (2 samples from the tibia interface, 2 samples from the talar interface, 1 sample from the capsule).
- The additional classification of the histologic samples according to the SLIM classification increases the quality of diagnosis and helps to understand the reason for TAR failure.
- Regardless of the type of infection and definitive treatment, the success rate after a complete implant removal is higher.
- Antibiotics can only support but not replace surgical treatment. Biofilm-active antibiotics are needed in patients with irrigation, debridement, and polyethylene exchange but implant retention. Biofilm-active antibiotics are also recommended to eradicate bacteria after the definitive surgical treatment with fusion or R-TAR.
- So far, no clear evidence exists to recommend either fusion or R-TAR after PJI.
- No conclusive data support a 1-stage revision over a 2-stage procedure. The clinical advantage of the 2-stage approach is the treatment according to the comprehensive intraoperative assessment, including results of histology and microbiology.

ACKNOWLEDGMENTS

The authors would like to thank Dr Anke Röser, Dr Andrej Tampuz, and Dr Vincent Krenn for their expertise and assistance throughout all aspects of our study and for their help in writing the article.

DISCLOSURE

The authors have nothing to disclose.

REFERENCES

1. Usuelli FG, Maccario C, Granata F, et al. Clinical and Radiological Outcomes of Transfibular Total Ankle Arthroplasty. Foot Ankle Int 2019;40(1):24–33.
2. Tiusanen H, Kormi S, Kohonen I, et al. Results of Trabecular-Metal Total Ankle Arthroplasties With Transfibular Approach. Foot Ankle Int 2020;41(4):411–8.
3. Yang HY, Wang SH, Lee KB. The HINTEGRA total ankle arthroplasty: functional outcomes and implant survivorship in 210 osteoarthritic ankles at a mean of 6.4 years. Bone Joint Lett J 2019;101-b(6):695–701.
4. Gougoulias N, Khanna A, Maffulli N. How successful are current ankle replacements?: a systematic review of the literature. Clin Orthop Relat Res 2010; 468(1):199–208.
5. Kessler B, Sendi P, Graber P, et al. Risk factors for periprosthetic ankle joint infection: a case-control study. J Bone Joint Surg Am 2012;94(20):1871–6.
6. Myerson MS, Shariff R, Zonno AJ. The management of infection following total ankle replacement: demographics and treatment. Foot Ankle Int 2014;35(9): 855–62.
7. Reuver JM, Dayerizadeh N, Burger B, et al. Total ankle replacement outcome in low volume centers: short-term followup. Foot Ankle Int 2010;31(12):1064–8.
8. Sambandam S, Serbin P, Riepen D, et al. Differences Between Total Ankle Replacement and Ankle Arthrodesis in Post-operative Complications and Reoperations at 30 Days and One Year. Cureus 2022;14(9):e28703.
9. Almutairi TA, Ragab KM, Elsayed SM, et al. Safety and efficacy of total ankle arthroplasty versus ankle arthrodesis for ankle osteoarthritis: A systematic review and meta-analysis. Foot 2023;55:101980.
10. Raikin SM, Kane J, Ciminiello ME. Risk factors for incision-healing complications following total ankle arthroplasty. J Bone Joint Surg Am 2010;92(12):2150–5.
11. Althoff A, Cancienne JM, Cooper MT, et al. Patient-Related Risk Factors for Periprosthetic Ankle Joint Infection: An Analysis of 6977 Total Ankle Arthroplasties. J Foot Ankle Surg 2018;57(2):269–72.
12. Lampley A, Gross CE, Green CL, et al. Association of Cigarette Use and Complication Rates and Outcomes Following Total Ankle Arthroplasty. Foot Ankle Int 2016;37(10):1052–9.
13. Patton D, Kiewiet N, Brage M. Infected total ankle arthroplasty: risk factors and treatment options. Foot Ankle Int 2015;36(6):626–34.
14. Schipper ON, Jiang JJ, Chen L, et al. Effect of diabetes mellitus on perioperative complications and hospital outcomes after ankle arthrodesis and total ankle arthroplasty. Foot Ankle Int 2015;36(3):258–67.
15. Gross CE, Green CL, DeOrio JK, et al. Impact of Diabetes on Outcome of Total Ankle Replacement. Foot Ankle Int 2015;36(10):1144–9.
16. Smyth NA, Kennedy JG, Parvizi J, et al. Risk factors for periprosthetic joint infection following total ankle replacement. Foot Ankle Surg 2020;26(5):591–5.
17. Zhang Z, Chien BY, Noori N, et al. Application of the Mayo Periprosthetic Joint Infection Risk Score for Total Ankle Arthroplasty. Foot Ankle Int 2023. https://doi.org/10.1177/10711007231157697. 10711007231157697.
18. Li C, Renz N, Trampuz A. Management of Periprosthetic Joint Infection. Hip Pelvis 2018;30(3):138–46.
19. Gellert M, Hardt S, Koder K, et al. Biofilm-active antibiotic treatment improves the outcome of knee periprosthetic joint infection: Results from a 6-year prospective cohort study. Int J Antimicrob Agents 2020;55(4):105904.

20. Osmon DR, Berbari EF, Berendt AR, et al. Diagnosis and management of prosthetic joint infection: clinical practice guidelines by the Infectious Diseases Society of America. Clin Infect Dis 2013;56(1):e1–25.

21. Muller S, Walther M, Roser A, et al. Endoprosthesis failure in the ankle joint : Histopathological diagnostics and classification. Orthopä 2017;46(3):234–41. Endoprothesenversagen im oberen Sprunggelenk : Histopathologische Diagnostik und Klassifikation.

22. Krenn V, Morawietz L, Perino G, et al. Revised histopathological consensus classification of joint implant related pathology. Pathol Res Pract 2014;210(12):779–86.

23. Krenn VT, Liebisch M, Kölbel B, et al. CD15 focus score: Infection diagnosis and stratification into low-virulence and high-virulence microbial pathogens in periprosthetic joint infection. Pathol Res Pract 2017;213(5):541–7.

24. Ruppert M, Theiss C, Knoss P, et al. Histopathological, immunohistochemical criteria and confocal laser-scanning data of arthrofibrosis. Pathol Res Pract 2013;209(11):681–8.

25. Richter D, Krahenbuhl N, Susdorf R, et al. What Are the Indications for Implant Revision in Three-component Total Ankle Arthroplasty? Clin Orthop Relat Res 2021;479(3):601–9.

26. Diniz SE, Ribau A, Vinha A, et al. Simple and inexpensive synovial fluid biomarkers for the diagnosis of prosthetic joint infection according to the new EBJIS definition. J Bone Jt Infect 2023;8(2):109–18.

27. Zheng QY, Ren P, Cheng L, et al. Leukocyte Esterase Strip Quantitative Detection Based on RGB Photometry is a Probable Method to Diagnose Periprosthetic Joint Infection: An Exploratory Study. Orthop Surg 2023;15(4):983–92.

28. Haertle M, Kolbeck L, Macke C, et al. Diagnostic Accuracy for Periprosthetic Joint Infection Does Not Improve by a Combined Use of Glucose and Leukocyte Esterase Strip Reading as Diagnostic Parameters. J Clin Med 2022;11(11). https://doi.org/10.3390/jcm11112979.

29. de Cesar Netto C, Fonseca LF, Fritz B, et al. Metal artifact reduction MRI of total ankle arthroplasty implants. Eur Radiol 2018;28(5):2216–27.

30. Renz N, Cabric S, Janz V, et al. [Sonication in the diagnosis of periprosthetic infections : Significance and practical implementation]. Orthopä 2015;44(12):942–5. Sonikation in der Diagnostik periprothetischer Infektionen : Stellenwert und praktische Umsetzung.

31. Achermann Y, Vogt M, Leunig M, et al. Improved diagnosis of periprosthetic joint infection by multiplex PCR of sonication fluid from removed implants. J Clin Microbiol 2010;48(4):1208–14.

32. Beguiristain I, Henriquez L, Sancho I, et al. Direct Prosthetic Joint Infection Diagnosis from Sonication Fluid Inoculated in Blood Culture Bottles by Direct MALDI-TOF Mass Spectrometry. Diagnostics 2023;13(5). https://doi.org/10.3390/diagnostics13050942.

33. Barrack RL, Aggarwal A, Burnett RS, et al. The fate of the unexpected positive intraoperative cultures after revision total knee arthroplasty. J Arthroplasty 2007;22(6 Suppl 2):94–9.

34. Jacobs AME, Benard M, Meis JF, et al. The unsuspected prosthetic joint infection : incidence and consequences of positive intra-operative cultures in presumed aseptic knee and hip revisions. Bone Joint Lett J 2017;99-B(11):1482–9.

35. Fuchs D. Should Culture Samples Be Taken During All Revision Total Ankle Arthroplasty (TAA)? Foot Ankle Int 2019;40(1_suppl):31S–2S.

36. Pfahl K, Roser A, Gottschalk O, et al. Common bacteria and treatment options for the acute and chronic infection of the total ankle arthroplasty. Foot Ankle Surg 2022;28(7):1008–13.
37. Lachman JR, Ramos JA, DeOrio JK, et al. Outcomes of Acute Hematogenous Periprosthetic Joint Infection in Total Ankle Arthroplasty Treated With Irrigation, Debridement, and Polyethylene Exchange. Foot Ankle Int 2018;39(11):1266–71.
38. Pfahl K, Roser A, Eder J, et al. Outcomes of Salvage Procedures for Failed Total Ankle Arthroplasty. Foot Ankle Int 2023. https://doi.org/10.1177/1071100723115 6426. 10711007231156426.
39. Tande AJ, Patel R. Prosthetic joint infection. Clin Microbiol Rev 2014;27(2): 302–45.
40. Rottier W, Seidelman J, Wouthuyzen-Bakker M. Antimicrobial treatment of patients with a periprosthetic joint infection: basic principles. Arthroplasty 2023; 5(1):10.
41. Beldman M, Lowik C, Soriano A, et al. Correction to: If, When, and How to Use Rifampin in Acute Staphylococcal Periprosthetic Joint Infections, a Multicentre Observational Study. Clin Infect Dis 2022;74(10):1890.
42. Le Vavasseur B, Zeller V. Antibiotic Therapy for Prosthetic Joint Infections: An Overview. Antibiotics (Basel) 2022;11(4). https://doi.org/10.3390/antibiotics11040486.
43. Li HK, Rombach I, Zambellas R, et al. Oral versus Intravenous Antibiotics for Bone and Joint Infection. N Engl J Med 2019;380(5):425–36.
44. Trampuz A, Renz N, Trebse R. Pocket guide to diagnosis & treatment of periprosthetic joint infection (PJI). Pro-Implant Foundation; 2023. Available at: https://pro-implant.org/tools/pocket-guide. Accessed April 22, 2023.
45. Renz N, Mudrovcic S, Perka C, et al. Orthopedic implant-associated infections caused by Cutibacterium spp. - A remaining diagnostic challenge. PLoS One 2018;13(8):e0202639.
46. Goud AL, Harlianto NI, Ezzafzafi S, et al. Reinfection rates after one- and two-stage revision surgery for hip and knee arthroplasty: a systematic review and meta-analysis. Arch Orthop Trauma Surg 2023;143(2):829–38.
47. D'Errico M, Morelli I, Castellini G, et al. Is debridement really the best we can do for periprosthetic joint infections following total ankle replacements? A systematic review and meta-analysis. Foot Ankle Surg 2022;28(6):697–708.
48. Kessler B, Knupp M, Graber P, et al. The treatment and outcome of periprosthetic infection of the ankle: a single cohort-centre experience of 34 cases. Bone Joint Lett J 2014;96-b(6):772–7.

Complications in Total Ankle Replacement

Joris P.S. Hermus, MD

KEYWORDS

• Total ankle replacement • Complications • Risk factors • Patient selection

KEY POINTS

• TARVA study shows no superiority between ankle arthrodesis and total ankle replacement.
• Defining complication is necessary to have accurate registration of complications.
• Complications with highest reported pooled incidence were intraoperative fracture 6% (95% CI 4%–8%) (GRADE very low) and impingement 6% (95% CI 4%–8%) (GRADE low), respectively.
• The risk of complications is much higher during the learning curve of a total ankle replacement.
• Lucency or cyst formation around the talar component was observed more frequently in mobile-bearing total ankle replacements.

INTRODUCTION

The debate between ankle arthrodesis and total ankle replacement for patients with end-stage arthritis of the ankle joint is an ongoing topic in orthopedic surgery.

Ankle arthrodesis, or fusion, has been the traditional treatment for ankle arthritis. It involves fusing the bones of the ankle joint together, eliminating the joint and creating a solid bony union. Arthrodesis is effective in reducing pain in the ankle, but it results in a loss of ankle motion. This can increase the load on adjacent joints, such as the subtalar joint, which may lead to accelerated degeneration and arthritis in those joints over time.[1–3]

Total ankle arthroplasty, on the other hand, involves replacing the arthritic ankle joint with a prosthetic implant. This allows for preservation of some degree of ankle motion and potentially more normal gait patterns compared with ankle fusion.[4] Total ankle replacement aims to provide pain relief while maintaining or restoring joint function.

The total ankle replacement versus ankle arthrodesis (TARVA) study, which compared total ankle replacement to ankle fusion, did not find clear superiority of either procedure. However, a post-hoc analysis of the study showed that the fixed-bearing total ankle

Maastricht University Medical Center +, Research School CAPHRI, Department Orthopaedic Surgery, P. Debyelaan 25, Maastricht 6229 HX, the Netherlands
E-mail address: j.hermus@mumc.nl

Foot Ankle Clin N Am 29 (2024) 157–163
https://doi.org/10.1016/j.fcl.2023.08.007
1083-7515/24/© 2023 Elsevier Inc. All rights reserved.

replacement resulted in significantly lower Manchester-Oxford Foot and Ankle Questionnaire (MOXFQ) scores compared with ankle arthrodesis and mobile-bearing total ankle replacement at 52 weeks.[5] This suggests that fixed-bearing total ankle replacement may provide better functional outcomes in the short term.

It is important to note that the TARVA study had a relatively short follow-up period of 1 year, which may limit the ability to assess long-term outcomes and complications of the procedures. Long-term studies with extended follow-up are needed to evaluate the durability and effectiveness of both ankle arthrodesis and total ankle arthroplasty.

Ultimately, the choice between ankle arthrodesis and total ankle arthroplasty depends on various factors, including the patient's age, activity level, overall health, severity of arthritis, and surgeon expertise. It is crucial for patients to have a thorough discussion with their orthopedic surgeon to understand the potential risks, benefits, and expected outcomes of each procedure before making a decision.

Defining What Is a Complication?

The definition of a complication is debatable. Ricketts and colleagues emphasized that there needs to be some clarity about the definition of a complication. The National Health Service defined a complication as any less than perfect outcome that increases the cost of treatment.[6] Sokol and Wilson defined a complication as any undesirable, unintended, and direct result of the ankle replacement.[7]

According to Mahmoud and colleagues' study, adverse events related to total ankle replacement are defined as unintended injuries or complications resulting from medical management that cause measurable disability, prolonged hospital stay, or even death.[8] It is important to note that not all adverse events are reported as complications, such as delayed wound healing. They found that 8.33% of the 648 reports in the Manufacturer and User Facility Device Experience database were not able to ascertain the specific complication or adverse event.

On the other hand, Van der Griend and colleagues emphasize the importance of distinguishing complications that require reoperation, not only in terms of numbers but also types.[9] This suggests that not all complications may necessitate reoperation, and it is crucial to understand the specific complications that lead to subsequent surgical interventions.

Glazebrook and colleagues proposed a more detailed classification based on the chance of failure.[10]

Low grade: Very unlikely to cause TAA failure

1. Intraoperative bone fracture
2. Wound healing problems

Medium grade: Leads to failure less than 50% of the time

1. Technical error
2. Subsidence
3. Postoperative bone fracture

High grade: Leads to failure greater than 50% of the time

1. Deep infection
2. Aseptic loosening
3. Implant failure

By categorizing adverse events and complications and understanding the ones that require reoperation, health care professionals and researchers can gain a better understanding of the risks and outcomes associated with total ankle replacement.

This information can ultimately contribute to improved management and decision-making related to this procedure.

Which Complications Can Occur in Total Ankle Replacement Surgery

Pubmed search found six English-written meta-analyses, which solely orientated on complications in total ankle replacement. In our own meta-analysis, we have reported the 10 most reported complications according the classification by Glazebrook: deep infection 2% (95% CI 1%–2% in 221 events in 12,963 ankles, 77 studies), aseptic loosening 5% (95% CI 3%–6% in 486 events in 9425 ankles), instability 2% (95% CI 1%–4% in 103 events in 3297 ankles, 23 studies), postoperative fracture 3% (95% CI 2%–3% in 437 events in 6388 ankles, 56 studies), component subsidence 4% (95% CI 2%–6% in 154 events in 3915 ankles, 37 studies), ongoing pain 4% (95% CI 3%–6% in 396 events in 5794 ankles, 45 studies), postoperative malalignment or deformity 4% (95% CI 3%–6% in180 events in 4936 ankles, 38 studies, 71 studies), impingement 6% (95% CI 4%–8% in 333 events in 5203 ankles, 47 studies), wound healing problems 4% (95% CI 3%–6% in 443 events in 7988 ankles, 61 studies), and intraoperative fracture 6% (95% CI 4%–8% in 348 events in 6100 ankles, 64 studies).[11] Complications with highest reported pooled incidence were intraoperative fracture 6% (95% CI 4%–8%) (GRADE very low) and impingement 6% (95% CI 4%–8%) (GRADE low), respectively. Impingement could be prevented by prophylactic widening of the medial and lateral gutters to diminish the prevalence of impingement.[12] Najefi and colleagues suggests that impingement could be caused by component malrotation.[13]

Most intraoperative fractures are iatrogenic, associated with inadequate exposure by the jig itself or size of the resection guide, together with inadvertent use of the saw blade.[14] Lazarides and colleagues suggests that all periprosthetic total ankle replacement fractures need to fixate.[15]

Jennison and colleagues reported a meta-analysis exclusively on thromboembolic events in total ankle replacements.[16] The incidence of reported postoperative DVT was 0.07% (95% CI 0.001%–0.59% in 81 events in 30,829 ankles, 18 studies). The pooled risk of a patient suffering a postoperative pulmonary was 0.01% (95% CI 0.001%–0.03% in 55 events in 28,335 ankles, 8 studies).

Is It Justified to Perform Ankle Replacement Surgery When There Is a High Risk of Complications and a Failure Rate?

Fanelli and colleagues performed a meta-analysis where they compared 5448 total ankle replacements with 13,175 ankle arthrodesis with a mean follow-up of 42.3 ± 16.8 months.[17] No significant differences were found in complication rate between total ankle replacement and ankle arthrodesis (OR 0.936, 95% CI 0.826–1.060; I2 = 87.44). Patient undergoing a total ankle replacement did not have a higher risk of reoperation for all causes compared with patients having an ankle arthrodesis (OR 1.720, 95% CI 0.892–3.316; I2 = 77.65).

Goldberg and colleagues performed a randomized clinical trial comparing the results of the total ankle replacement and ankle arthrodesis group.[5] The total ankle replacement group had a higher incidence of wound healing complications (13.8% compared with 5.5% in the ankle arthrodesis group). In addition, nerve injuries were more prevalent in the total ankle replacement group compared with the ankle arthrodesis group (4.3% vs <1%). On the other hand, thromboembolic events (such as blood clots) were less common in the total ankle replacement group (3%) compared with the ankle arthrodesis group (5%). It is clear that nonunions only occurred in the ankle arthrodesis group (11.3%). Nonetheless, there was no significant difference found in the improved MOXFQ-W/S scores between the total ankle replacement group and the ankle arthrodesis group at 52 weeks postoperatively. A post-hoc analysis showed better outcomes in the fixed-bearing total ankle replacement compared with the ankle arthrodesis at 52 weeks of follow-up.

How Can We Minimize the Risk of Complications?

While reporting our results with the CCI total ankle replacement system, we noted that all our perioperative complications in our first 30 ankle replacements.[18] Schimmel and colleagues advised in their article that stricter patient selection for total ankle replacement especially during the first 50 total ankle replacements.[19] During the learning curve period, careful surgical indications and surgeries are desired. A meta-analysis of 25 articles by Simonson and colleagues reports the risk of complications during the learning curve of a total ankle replacement.[20] A total of 1085 complications occurred during their learning curve in 2453 total ankle replacements, yielding an overall incidence of complications of 44.2%. In addition, Kurokawa and colleagues advised that involving experienced surgeons as assistants can lead to favorable results, even when the primary surgeon lacks experience.[21] This further supports the notion that the involvement of experienced surgeons during the learning curve can help mitigate complications and improve outcomes.

Albright and colleagues found in their meta-analysis that inpatient surgery had a fivefold higher risk of short-term complications compared with outpatient surgery.[22] On the other hand, Tedder and colleagues reported that their inpatient population was significantly older, had longer operative times, and higher rates of diabetes. Nonetheless, it could suggest that a healthy patient without comorbidity can be treated outpatient for total ankle replacement.[23]

Are There Implant-Related Factors at Risk for Complications?

The randomized clinical trial by Goldberg and colleagues showed with a post-hoc analysis that the fixed-bearing total ankle replacement resulted in significantly lower MOXFQ scores compared with ankle arthrodesis and mobile-bearing total ankle replacement at 52 weeks.[5] Nunley and colleagues performed a randomized clinical trial comparing the outcomes between mobile- and fixed-bearing total ankle replacement with an average follow-up of 4.5 years.[24] Visual analogue scale (VAS), 36-item short form health survey (SF-36), foot and ankle disability index (FADI), short musculoskeletal function assessment (SMFA), and American Orthopedic Foot and Ankle Society (AOFAS) ankle-hindfoot scores demonstrated no statistically significant differences between the mobile bearing- and fixed-bearing total ankle replacement cohorts. Although lucency or cyst around the talar component was observed more frequently in the mobile bearing group ($P = .01$). Malalignment occurred also more significantly in the mobile-bearing group as well for the tibial as the talar component. Reoperations were also performed more often in the mobile bearing group, with most procedures being to relieve impingement or treat cysts. Arcângelo and colleagues confirmed similar results in their meta-analysis that nonanatomic, mobile-bearing, hydroxyapatite-coated and non-tibial-stemmed total ankle replacements were positively associated with more periprosthetic bone cysts (430 developed periprosthetic cystic osteolysis in 2430 total ankle replacements in 21 articles).[25]

Are There Patient-Related Factors at Risk for Complications?

Most articles relate the patient-related factors to failures instead of complications. So, the Swedish register, there was a significantly higher risk of failure in case of patients (especially women) younger than 60 years of age with osteoarthritis or post-traumatic arthritis.[26] Our own Dutch Arthroplasty Register study showed that patients with prior osteochondral defect (OCD) surgery seem to have a higher risk for implant failure and a higher body mass index (BMI) and a lower age were also determined as a risk factor for implant failure.[27]

Althoff and colleagues performed a cohort study of 6977 patients. 294 patients (4%) had the diagnosis of, or had undergone a procedure for, periprosthetic joint infection. Risk factors found for periprosthetic joint infection included age less than 65 years (OR 1.44; $P = .036$), body mass index less than 19 kg/m^2 (OR 3.35; $P = .013$), body mass index greater than 30 kg/m^2 (OR 1.49; $P = .034$), tobacco use (OR 1.59; $P = .002$), diabetes mellitus (OR 1.36; $P = .017$), inflammatory arthritis (OR 2.38; $P < .0001$), peripheral vascular disease (OR 1.64; $P < .0001$), chronic lung disease (OR 1.37; $P = .022$), and hypothyroidism (OR 1.32; $P = .022$). Most reported patient-related risk factors for complications were concerning periprosthetic joint infection and wound problems.[28]

Recently, Lewis and colleagues propose a five-factor-modified frailty index as a predictor of complications following total ankle replacement.[29] The modified 5-item frailty index (mFI-5) is composed of five risk factors: history of diabetes mellitus, history of hypertension, history of congestive heart failure (with an exacerbation within 30 days before surgery), history of severe chronic obstructive pulmonary disease (COPD) or current pneumonia, and nonindependent functional status (requiring some or complete assistance with activities of daily living).

Patients with an mFI-5 score of 0 had a wound complication rate of 0.24%. In comparison, patients with an mFI-5 score of $\geq$2 had a higher wound complication rate of 1.55%. Patients with an mFI-5 score of 0 had a complication rate of 5.24%, whereas those with an mFI-5 score of $\geq$2 had a significantly higher complication rate of 19.38%. This suggests that patients with higher frailty scores are more likely to experience complications.

SUMMARY

Total ankle replacement is a proven effective procedure to relief pain and to preserve function in end-stage ankle arthritis. The complications rate of total ankle replacement is highly variable across studies. Multiple factors, such as the surgeon's experience, patient's specific health factors, and activity pattern, could be additional determinants as a risk factor for complications in total ankle replacement. Awareness of these complications which occur in total ankle replacement is necessary, to achieve a decrease in complication rates in total ankle replacement surgery. Further research should focus on a more thorough patient selection to reducing the complication of total ankle replacements.

CLINICS CARE POINTS

- Intraoperative fracture and impingements are the most reported complications in total ankle replacement.

- Rotation of the component could be a reason for impingement.

- A more thorough patient selection is necessary to reduce he complication rate of total ankle replacements.

DISCLOSURE

J.P.S. Hermus; Board member/committee appointments for a society (The following conflicts were disclosed) European Foot and Ankle Society & Dutch Foot and Ankle Society.

REFERENCES

1. Heckmann N, Bradley A, Sivasundaram L, et al. Effect of insurance on rates of total ankle arthroplasty versus arthrodesis for tibiotalar osteoarthritis. Foot Ankle Int 2017;38:133–9.
2. Michael JM, Golshani A, Gargac S, et al. Biomechanics of the ankle joint and clinical outcomes of total ankle replacement. J Mech Behav Biomed Mater 2008;1(4):276–94.
3. Schmid T, Krause FG. Conservative treatment of asymmetric ankle osteoarthritis. Foot Ankle Clin 2013;18(3):437–48.
4. Deleu PA, Besse JL, Naaim A, et al. Change in gait biomechanics after total ankle replacement and ankle arthrodesis: a systematic review and meta-analysis. Clin Biomech 2020;73:213–25.
5. Goldberg AJ, Chowdhury K, Bordea E, et al, TARVA Study Group. Total ankle replacement versus arthrodesis for end-stage ankle osteoarthritis: a randomized controlled trial. Ann Intern Med 2022;175(12):1648–57.
6. Ricketts D, Rogers RA, Roper T, et al. Recognising and dealing with complications in orthopaedic surgery. Ann R Coll Surg Engl 2017;99(3):185–8.
7. Sokol DK, Wilson J. What is a surgical complication? World J Surg 2008;32(6):942–4.
8. Mahmoud K, Metikala S, O'Connor KM, et al. Adverse events related to total ankle replacement devices: an analysis of reports to the United States Food and Drug Administration. Int Orthop 2021;45(9):2307–12.
9. Vander Griend RA, Younger ASE, Buedts K, et al. Total ankle arthroplasty: minimum follow-up policy for reporting results and guidelines for reporting problems and complications resulting in reoperations. Foot Ankle Int 2017;38(7):703–4.
10. Glazebrook MA, Arsenault K, Dunbar M. Evidence-based classification of complications in total ankle arthroplasty. Foot Ankle Int 2009;30(10):945–9.
11. Hermus JP, Voesenek JA, van Gansewinkel EHE, et al. Complications following total ankle arthroplasty: a systematic literature review and meta-analysis. Foot Ankle Surg 2022;28(8):1183–93.
12. Schuberth JM, Babu NS, Richey JM, et al. Gutter impingement after total ankle arthroplasty. Foot Ankle Int 2013;34(3):329–37.
13. Najefi AA, Ghani Y, Goldberg A. Role of rotation in total ankle replacement. Foot Ankle Int 2019;40(12):1358–67.
14. Manegold S, Haas NP, Manegold S, et al. Peri-prosthetic fractures in total ankle replacement: classification system and treatment algorithm. J Bone Jt Surg Am 2013;95:815–20.
15. Lazarides AL, Vovos TJ, Reddy GB, et al. Algorithm for management of periprosthetic ankle fractures. Foot Ankle Int 2019;40(6):615–21.
16. Jennison T, Taher S, Ukoumunne O, et al. Pulmonary embolism, mortality, and medical complications following a total ankle replacement: a systematic review and meta-analysis. Foot Ankle Int 2023;44(3):223–31.
17. Fanelli D, Mercurio M, Castioni D, et al. End-stage ankle osteoarthritis: arthroplasty offers better quality of life than arthrodesis with similar complication and re-operation rates-an updated meta-analysis of comparative studies. Int Orthop 2021;45(9):2177–91.
18. Hermus JPS, van Kuijk SM, Witlox MA, et al. Alignment of CCI total ankle replacements in relation to midterm functional outcome and complication incidence. J Foot Ankle Res 2023;16(1):34.

19. Schimmel JJ, Walschot LH, Louwerens JW. Comparison of the short-term results of the first and last 50 Scandinavian total ankle replacements: assessment of the learning curve in a consecutive series. Foot Ankle Int 2014;35(4):326–33.
20. Simonson DC, Roukis TS. Incidence of complications during the surgeon learning curve period for primary total ankle replacement: a systematic review. Clin Podiatr Med Surg 2015;32(4):473–82.
21. Kurokawa H, Taniguchi A, Miyamoto T, et al. What is the best way for an inexperienced surgeon to learn total anklearthroplasty? J Orthop Sci 2023;28(4):849–52.
22. Albright RH, Rodela RJ, Nabili P, et al. Complication rates following total ankle arthroplasty in inpatient versus outpatient populations: a systematic review & meta-analysis. J Foot Ankle Surg 2021;60(1):61–6.
23. Tedder C, DeBell H, Dix D, et al. Comparative analysis of short-term postoperative complications in outpatient versus inpatient total ankle arthroplasty: a database study. J Foot Ankle Surg 2019;58(1):23–6.
24. Nunley JA, Adams SB, Easley ME, et al. Prospective randomized trial comparing mobile-bearing and fixed-bearing total ankle replacement. Foot Ankle Int 2019; 40(11):1239–48.
25. Arcângelo J, Guerra-Pinto F, Pinto A, et al. Peri-prosthetic bone cysts after total ankle replacement. A systematic review and meta-analysis. Foot Ankle Surg 2019;25(2):96–105.
26. Henricson A, Nilsson JÅ, Carlsson A. 10-year survival of total ankle arthroplasties: a report on 780 cases from the Swedish Ankle Register. Acta Orthop 2011;82(6): 655–9.
27. Hermus JPS, van Kuijk SMJ, Spekenbrink-Spooren A, et al. Risk factors for total ankle arthroplasty failure: a Dutch arthroplasty register study. Foot Ankle Surg 2022;28(7):883–6.
28. Althoff A, Cancienne JM, Cooper MT, et al. Patient-related risk factors for peri-prosthetic ankle joint infection: an analysis of 6977 total ankle arthroplasties. J Foot Ankle Surg 2018;57(2):269–72.
29. Lewis LK, Jupiter DC, Panchbhavi VK, et al. Five-factor modified frailty index as a predictor of complications following total ankle arthroplasty. Foot Ankle Spec 2023. 19386400231169368. https://journals.sagepub.com/doi/epub/10.1177/19386400231169368.

Outcomes of Conversion of Ankle Fusion to Total Ankle Arthroplasty

Christopher Traynor, MD[a,b], J. Chris Coetzee, MD[a,b],*

KEYWORDS

- Failed ankle fusion • Adjacent joint arthritis • Malunion • Nonunion
- Conversion of an ankle fusion

KEY POINTS

- The historical standard for treating end-stage ankle arthritis has been ankle arthrodesis.
- Issues such as adjacent joint arthritis, altered gait mechanics, activity limitations, non-unions, and malalignment can all cause pain, discomfort, and functional limitations for patients.
- The management of a painful ankle following an ankle fusion can be a complicated and difficult undertaking.
- One potential solution is converting the ankle fusion to total ankle arthroplasty. This can help improve pain, function, and motion in patients.

INTRODUCTION

The historical standard for treating end-stage ankle arthritis has been ankle arthrodesis. Done correctly, it is a durable, pain-relieving procedure. However, ankle fusions do not come without complications. Issues such as adjacent joint arthritis, altered gait mechanics, activity limitations, nonunions, and malalignment can all cause pain, discomfort, and functional limitations for patients.[1–4] Following a tibiotalar arthrodesis, abnormal loads are placed on surrounding joints resulting in higher rates of adjacent joint arthritis.[4–7] Initially, it is felt that the loss of motion through the ankle joint is compensated through increased motion at the talonavicular (TN) and subtalar (ST) joints. However, this is an abnormal, incongruent motion that can lead to early, progressive joint degeneration. The management of a painful ankle following an ankle fusion can be a complicated and difficult undertaking. One potential solution is converting the ankle fusion to total ankle arthroplasty (TAA). This can help improve pain, function, and motion in patients.[8–14]

^a Twin Cities Orthopedics, Minneapolis, MN, USA; ^b Twin Cities Orthopedics, 2700 Vikings Circle, Eagan, MN 55121, USA
* Corresponding author.
E-mail address: jcc@tcomn.com

Foot Ankle Clin N Am 29 (2024) 165–170
https://doi.org/10.1016/j.fcl.2023.08.008
1083-7515/24/© 2023 Elsevier Inc. All rights reserved.

foot.theclinics.com

BACKGROUND

Pain following ankle arthrodesis is a challenging clinical picture. It is first important to distinguish if the pain has been present since the fusion or if it presented after a period of relative comfort. If the pain has been persistent since the fusion, potential sources include nonunion, malunion, or infection. Imaging and lab tests should be completed to help elucidate the cause. When nonsurgical care fails, surgical considerations include revision arthrodesis or adjacent joint arthrodesis versus arthrodesis takedown and insertion of TAA.

If discomfort arises after an interval of relative painlessness, the most common reason is adjacent joint arthritis. Adjacent joint degeneration is a known long-term complication of tibiotalar arthrodesis. It most commonly presents in the ST joint but can affect the TN joint and surrounding hindfoot and midfoot joints as well.[4–7] Imaging and selective injections can help to identify symptomatic adjacent joints. Surgery should be considered when nonoperative care has been exhausted. Fusion of the involved joints results in a much stiffer hindfoot and ankle, notably as the ST joint is most involved. It is well-known that pantalar fusions often leave patients dissatisfied and should be reserved as a salvage option.[15] Ankle fusion takedown with TAA alongside concomitant or staged adjacent joint fusion serves as a viable alternative. We feel that simultaneous fusion of adjacent joints should be avoided unless absolutely necessary. There runs a risk of devascularization of the talus, and many patients may improve symptomatically simply by restoration of ankle range of motion (ROM) and reduction of adjacent joint loading.[12]

Common indications for ankle fusion takedown with conversion to TAA include painful malunion, nonunion, or painful osteoarthritis of adjacent joints following ankle fusion. Although no clear guidelines exist, patients often excluded include those with peripheral neuropathy, an unknown source of pain, neurovascular compromise, the absence of malleoli secondary to or prior to the fusion technique, and a history of infection.[9–14]

PROCEDURAL APPROACH

- Position the patient supine with a bump under the operative hip.
- A nonsterile thigh tourniquet is placed and inflated to 300 mm Hg following limb exsanguination.
- A 12 to 14 cm longitudinal anterior approach should be used, although it can be modified for previous skin incisions.
- Anteroposterior and lateral radiographs can be used to identify the original joint line. The original joint line is about 10 mm distal to the epiphyseal scar and it can act as a guide (**Fig. 1**).
- Insert a pin in the anterior tibial tuberosity and place an external tibial guide.
- Attach a cutting jig and again confirm joint level with fluoroscopy.
- Pins can be utilized to protect the medial and lateral malleoli from the oscillating saw.
- The initial tibial cut should be perpendicular to the long axis of the tibia and just distal to the epiphyseal scar.
- The vertical medial and lateral cuts can be made with a reciprocating saw in line the medial and lateral gutters. These again should be carefully determined utilizing fluoroscopy.
- In a well-positioned fusion, the talar cut should be placed 12 to 14 mm distal to the tibial cut.
- If there is a coronal plane deformity, this can be corrected by holding the hindfoot in neutral position and paralleling the tibial and talar cuts.

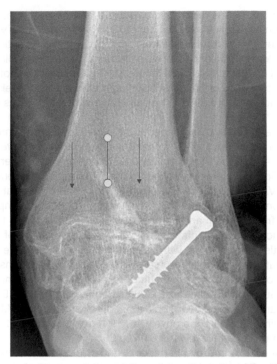

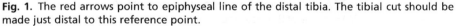

Fig. 1. The red arrows point to epiphyseal line of the distal tibia. The tibial cut should be made just distal to this reference point.

- Ensure the joint line and gutters are adequately debrided from the bone and soft tissue.
- Utilize trials to assess stability and help with sizing.
- Place final components and verify positioning with fluoroscopy.
- Achilles tendon lengthening, lateral or medial ligament release, or reconstructions can be completed at this time.
- Again, adjacent joint fusions (TN and ST joints) should only be done with severe cases to avoid talar devascularization.

POSTOPERATIVE CARE

Postoperatively, patients should be splinted for the first 2 weeks allowing 50% weight-bearing. Weeks 2 to 6, the patient can be transitioned in the controlled ankle movement boot allowing continued 50% weight-bearing. ROM exercises when seated should be encouraged. Physical therapy and progression to full weight-bearing can be initiated at 6 weeks postoperatively.

DISCUSSION AND OUTCOMES

Very little has been published on takedown of ankle fusions and conversion to TAA. Newton initially reported on 3 patients who underwent TAA in the setting of ankle fusion nonunion. All 3 implants failed, and he recommended against TAA in patients with a failed ankle fusion.[16] Modern implants and techniques, however, have borne better results.

Greisberg and colleagues reported on 19 ankle fusions converted to TAA in 18 patients with 39 months of follow-up. Ten out of 19 had no or mild pain with average ROM of 26°. They noted that all patients with a prior distal fibula resection did poorly and those without a clear source of pain pre-op did worse.[13] Similarly, Hintermann and colleagues reported on their series of 29 ankles in 27 patients. They noted an 83% satisfaction rate with only 10% of patients reporting continued pain levels greater than 3.0 on the visual analogue score (VAS). The patients' average ROM was noted to be 24.3° postoperatively.[14]

Even more recent data with larger series have demonstrated some improvement in most patients. In their series of 77 patients who underwent conversion of an ankle arthrodesis to TAA, Schuberth and colleagues determined that American Orthopaedic Foot and Ankle Society scores improved from a mean of 33 preoperatively to 75 postoperatively and VAS scores decreased from a mean of 8 preoperatively to 3 postoperatively. Additionally, they noted 88% of patients retained their implants an average of 8.6 years out from revision and had a mean ROM of 20.1° at 24 months postoperatively.[9] Our cohort of 51 patients was followed over an average of 4.2 years. We reported a high satisfaction number with patients reporting an average of 87.9 out of 100 possible on a patient satisfaction survey. Additionally, we demonstrated significant differences in most patient-reported outcome scores including the Veterans RAND 12 Item Health Survey physical scores (28.7 preoperatively to 38.9 postoperatively), the Ankle Osteoarthritis Scale (AOS) pain (55.9 preoperatively to 27.9 postoperatively) and AOS disability (61.7 preoperatively to 31.1 postoperatively). VAS scores also improved from a preoperative level of 64.5 to 29.4.[12]

Overall pain seems to improve in patients undergoing a takedown of ankle fusion with conversion to TAA.[9–14] However, residual pain persists. A recent metaanalysis notes an average VAS score of 2.5 postoperatively with no study noting results better than 1.8.[8] This is an important point when discussing postoperative expectations with our patients.

Improvement in ROM is arguably the most important functional outcome from an ankle fusion takedown. Increased ROM reduces adject joint stresses and can improve quality of life. All studies have demonstrated improvement in ROM for their cohorts. Average ROM at final follow-up ranges from 20.1° to 29.6°.[9,12] This likely leads to better gait mechanics and overall mobility. **Fig. 2** demonstrates typical postoperative motion from an ankle fusion takedown to TAA.

Complication rates and severity of complications differ among studies. Known complications include fracture, malalignment, arthrofibrosis and impingement, wound complications, implant loosening, and infection. Overall implant survival rates range

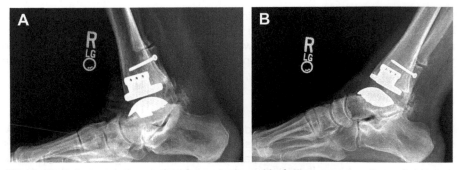

Fig. 2. (*A, B*) Postoperative motion from a prior ankle fusion nonunion that subsequently underwent conversion to total ankle arthroplasty.

from 2% to 42%. The Chu metaanalysis notes an overall TAA revision rate to be at 10.4%, a number they note is not dissimilar to primary TAA studies albiet with a shorter follow-up of only 62.8 months. The rates of transtibial amputation and TTC arthrodesis according to the Chu study are both at 2.3%.[8] Initial studies demonstrated relatively high rates of intraoperative malleolar fractures ranging from 9% to 43%.[10,13,14] In our most recent cohort, we only saw 1 medial malleolar fracture out of 51 patients.[12] Careful fusion takedown with judicious use of prophylactic fixation can help minimize malleolar fractures.

SUMMARY

Pain in the setting of a prior ankle fusion can be due to malunion or nonunion at the fusion versus adjacent joint degeneration. Ankle fusion takedown with conversion to TAA is a viable treatment option for these patients. It improves ROM and reduces pain in most patients. However, residual pain is a common occurrence with known complications including fracture, malalignment, arthrofibrosis and impingement, wound complications, implant loosening, and infection.

CLINICS CARE POINTS

- Pain following an ankle arthrodesis can be a challenging clinical picture.
- Pain at the fusion site is from nonunion or malunion and often has been present since the date of fusion.
- Pain that presents after a pain-free period most likely derives from adjacent joint disease, most commonly involving the ST joint.
- Indications for ankle fusion takedown with conversion to TAA include painful malunion, nonunion, or painful osteoarthritis of adjacent joints following ankle fusion.
- Exclusions include those with peripheral neuropathy, an unknown source of pain, neurovascular compromise, the absence of malleoli secondary to or prior to the fusion technique, and a history of infection.
- During surgery, utilize fluoroscopy judiciously.
- The former joint line can be found 10 mm distal to the epiphyseal scar.
- The tibial cut should be just distal the epiphyseal scar, the talar cut 12 to 14 mm distal to that
- Adjacent joint fusions should be avoided at the time of TAA if possible, to avoid talar devascularization
- Pain and ROM both tend to improve following surgery, although some level of pain is common following the procedure
- Common complications include fracture, malalignment, arthrofibrosis and impingement, wound complications, implant loosening, and infection

DISCLOSURE

J.C. Coetzee is a consultant for Smith and Nephew.

REFERENCES

1. Mazur JM, Schwartz E, Simon SR. Ankle arthrodesis. Long-term follow-up with gait analysis. J Bone Joint Surg Am 1979;61(7):964–75.

2. Muir DC, Amendola A, Saltzman CL. Long-term outcome of ankle arthrodesis. Foot Ankle Clin 2002;7(4):703–8.
3. Chalayon O, Wang B, Blankenhorn B, et al. Factors Affecting the Outcomes of Uncomplicated Primary Open Ankle Arthrodesis. Foot Ankle Int 2015;36(10): 1170–9.
4. Aaron AD. Ankle fusion: a retrospective review. Orthopedics 1990;13(11): 1249–54.
5. Ling JS, Smyth NA, Fraser EJ, et al. Investigating the relationship between ankle arthrodesis and adjacent-joint arthritis in the hindfoot: a systematic review. J Bone Joint Surg Am 2015;97(6):513–20.
6. Davis RJ, Millis MB. Ankle arthrodesis in the management of traumatic ankle arthrosis: a long-term retrospective study. J Trauma 1980;20(8):674–8.
7. Coester LM, Saltzman CL, Leupold J, et al. Long-term results following ankle arthrodesis for post-traumatic arthritis. J Bone Joint Surg Am 2001;83(2):219–28.
8. Chu AK, Wilson MD, Houng B, et al. Outcomes of Ankle Arthrodesis Conversion to Total Ankle Arthroplasty: A Systematic Review. J Foot Ankle Surg 2021;60(2): 362–7.
9. Schuberth JM, King CM, Jiang SF, et al. Takedown of Painful Ankle Arthrodesis to Total Ankle Arthroplasty: A Case Series of 77 Patients. J Foot Ankle Surg 2020; 59(3):535–40.
10. Pellegrini MJ, Schiff AP, Adams SB, et al. Conversion of Tibiotalar Arthrodesis to Total Ankle Arthroplasty. J Bone Joint Surg Am 2015;97(24):2004–13.
11. Preis M, Bailey T, Marchand LS, et al. Can a Three-Component Prosthesis be Used for Conversion of Painful Ankle Arthrodesis to Total Ankle Replacement? Clin Orthop Relat Res 2017;475(9):2283–94.
12. Lundeen AL, Raduan FC, Stone McGaver R, et al. Takedown of Ankle Fusions and Conversion to Total Ankle Replacements. Foot Ankle Int 2022;43(11):1402–9.
13. Greisberg J, Assal M, Flueckiger G, et al. Takedown of Ankle Fusion and Conversion to Total Ankle Replacement. Clin Orthop Relat Res 2004;424:80–8.
14. Hintermann B, Barg A, Knupp M, et al. Conversion of Painful Ankle Arthrodesis to Total Ankle Arthroplasty. Journal of Bone and Joint Surgery-American 2009;91(4): 850–8.
15. Acosta R, Ushiba J, Cracchiolo A. The results of a primary and staged pantalar arthrodesis and tibiotalocalcaneal arthrodesis in adult patients. Foot Ankle Int 2000;21(3):182–94.
16. Newton SE. Total ankle arthroplasty. Clinical study of fifty cases. J Bone Joint Surg Am 1982;64(1):104–11.

Outcomes of Revision Total Ankle Replacement

Bakur A. Jamjoom, BMBS, ChM, FRCS Orth, FRCS (T & O)[a],*,
Sunil Dhar, MBBS, MS, MCh Orth, FRCS Ed Orth[b]

KEYWORDS

- Total ankle arthroplasty • Total ankle replacement • Revision ankle arthroplasty
- Revision ankle replacement • Foot and ankle surgery • Functional outcome

KEY POINTS

- Revision total ankle arthroplasty (TAA) is an effective option for the treatment of failed primary TAA, more so as newer implants, improved instrumentation, and additive technologies become increasingly available.
- At median follow-up of 4 years, the median survival and reoperation rates were 86% and 16%, respectively.
- Significant postoperative improvements in patient-reported outcome measures were documented in 6 of 12 studies.
- The literature on the outcome of revision TAA is still limited in quantity and duration.

BACKGROUND

Over the last 3 decades, there has been considerable development in total ankle arthroplasty (TAA) with newer generations of prosthesis featuring better biomechanical designs, superior materials, and improved implantation techniques.[1–3] As a result, TAA is fast becoming the ideal treatment option for many patients with end-stage ankle arthritis, providing pain relief and preserving range of movement. The utilization rate of TAA in the United States saw a substantial rise between 1998 and 2010, going from 0.13 to 0.84 per 100,000 population.[4] Similarly, the total annual number of TAA procedures reported in the UK National Joint Registry increased significantly from 603 in 2013 to 1023 in 2022.[5]

Declarations: S. Dhar is a paid consultant and a member of the TAR design team for Stryker. NUH has received research funding from Wright Medical (Stryker) for portfolio management service of the Infinity implant.
[a] Leeds Teaching Hospitals, Chapel Allerton Hospital, Leeds LS7 4SA, UK; [b] Foot and Ankle Unit, Nottingham Elective Orthopaedics, Nottingham University Hospitals City Campus, Nottingham NG5 1PB, UK
* Corresponding author.
E-mail address: bakur.jamjoom@gmail.com

Foot Ankle Clin N Am 29 (2024) 171–184
https://doi.org/10.1016/j.fcl.2023.08.012
1083-7515/24/© 2023 Elsevier Inc. All rights reserved.

foot.theclinics.com

Despite substantial improvement in outcomes, survival rates for TAA are yet to equal those of hip and knee arthroplasties.[6] The survival rates for primary TAA have been reported as 81% to 93% at 5 years, 69% to 86% at 10 years, and 45.6% to 63.6% at 15 years.[2,3,6,7]

Given the increasing trend in primary TAA utilization[4,5] and its current rate of revision, it is inevitable that a large volume of failed TAAs will require action by foot and ankle surgeons in the future. In fact, it is estimated that between 3000 and 5000 failing ankle replacements will require treatment in the United Kingdom alone over the next 2 decades.[3,5]

The treatment of a failed TAA is a challenging endeavor, and the options include revision TAA, ankle arthrodesis,[1,8,9] ankle-hindfoot arthrodesis,[10,11] and amputation. Arthrodesis had been considered the favored procedure for the salvage of failed TAA but its variable functional outcomes have thrown doubt over this assertion.[1,8,9,12] Revision TAA is a complex operation that may have to deal with bone loss, deformity, and soft tissues challenges and often requires secondary procedures. It is affected by prosthesis design and instrumentation, along with the indication for revision and the experience of the surgeon.[13–15] Revision TAA has been associated with a higher risk of complications and worse outcomes when compared to primary TAA.[16–18] Recent advancements in implant design, surgical technique, and imaging planning capabilities are transforming the outcomes of revision TAA. At present, there is a paucity in the literature of the outcomes of revision TAA with most studies reporting short-term outcomes and only a limited number of cases. This study aims to provide an up-to-date overview of the current literature on the survival rates, clinical, and radiographic outcomes of revision TAA.

METHODS
Literature Search

To ensure comprehensive coverage of revision TAA in the update, a systematic literature review was conducted by searching various databases including PubMed, Medline, Embase, and the Cochrane Central Register of Controlled Trials in December 2022. A combination or part combination of relevant keywords including ankle, arthroplasty, replacement, prosthesis, total, revision, outcomes, results, and survival were used to filter the search results. The titles were evaluated, and the abstracts of eligible studies were examined. The full texts of potentially suitable articles were retrieved and evaluated. Additionally, the bibliography was reviewed for additional relevant articles.

The term "Revision TAA" has been used in the literature to describe several procedures that include exchange of 1 or more components, revision to an arthrodesis, or just implant removal.[14] For the purposes of this study, the authors have considered revision TAA to be the exchange of 1 or both tibial and/or talar components to another TAA implant. In most instances, this also includes the insert.

Eligibility Criteria

The inclusion criteria were articles that were published in the English language in the last decade (2013–2022) and reported patients who had undergone revision ankle arthroplasty as a treatment for failed primary TAA. The authors included articles that reported results of revision TAA and provided sufficient data relating to the cohorts' demographic, radiographic, and clinical outcomes with a minimum 2 year follow-up period. The authors excluded studies that focused on primary TAA,[19–21] studies that did not provide adequate data,[18,22] systematic reviews,[12,23–27] abstracts not published as full articles,[28–30] and articles that were published prior to 2013.[31]

Data Extraction

Data were extracted from the selected studies using a standardized form. The 2 authors performed this independently and compared the results to reduce extraction errors. Any discrepancies were discussed and resolved by consensus. Missing data were referred to not available. The following data were collected for each study: year of publication, study level of evidence (LOE), cohort's mean age and gender, indication for the revision, type of implant used in the revision, rates of infection, application of other procedures, reoperation, conversion to fusion, and survival. The authors also included the findings relating to the utilized patient-reported clinical outcome measures (PROMs): American Orthopaedic Foot and Ankle Society (AOFAS), Manchester-Oxford Foot Questionnaire (MOXFQ), Visual Analogue Score (VAS), Ankle Osteoarthritis Scale (AOS), EuroQol-5 Dimensions (EQ5D), Foot Function Index (FFI), Short Form 36 (SF-36), and Short Musculoskeletal Function Assessment (SMFA). Furthermore, the data collection entered all the radiographic outcomes measures reported in the various studies relating to alignment of components, osteolysis, subsidence, loosening, and heterotopic ossification (HO). The LOE of the various studies was extracted from the publication when mentioned; otherwise, the 2 authors independently assessed the methodological quality of the article and determined its LOE using the Oxford LOE Scale.[32]

Outcome Measures

The primary outcomes were the rates of reoperation and implant survival along with the results of the PROMs and radiographic outcomes.

Data Evaluation

The results for the rates of reoperation and implant survival were pooled, and the median (range) findings for all the studies were calculated. As a result of the variation in the clinical and radiographic methods of assessment between the various series, the analysis was descriptive and focused on stating all the significant or insignificant findings that were reported by the authors.

RESULTS
Study Selection and Cohort Characteristics

The literature research identified 12 studies that met the inclusion criteria and reported a total of 419 revision TAA patients.[3,8,13,16,17,33–39] The findings are summarized as follows:

- The median number of patients per study was 26 (ranging from 10–117).
- The median mean age of patients was 59 (ranging from 52–68) years, and the median percentage of female patients was 44% (ranging from 23%–71%).
- The median duration between the primary and revision TAA procedures was 72 (ranging from 22–94) months, as reported in 11 studies.
- The majority of revision TAA procedures were for aseptic complications (loosening, lysis, cysts, and so forth), with a median of 99% (ranging from 74%–100%).
- The median percentage of revision TAA procedures for infection was 1.5% (ranging from 0%–26%), with 1 study being graded as LOE-II.[16]
- Two studies were graded as LOE-III,[17,34] and the remaining 9 studies were graded as LOE-IV.
- The median duration of follow-up was 48 (ranging from 24–83) months.
- Patient characteristics for the various series are summarized in **Table 1**.

Table 1
Characteristics of the revision total ankle arthroplasty patients in the 12 selected studies

Author, Year	Number of Revised Ankles	Mean Age	Percent of Females	Indication for Revision		Timing of Revision (Months)	Follow-up (Months)	Study Level of Evidence
				Aseptic	Septic			
Jamjoom et al,[3] 2022	29	68	36%	100%	0%	88	40	IV
Jennison et al,[16] 2021	23	65	23%	74%	26%	NA	24	II
Behrens et al,[13] 2020	18	58	61%	89%	11%	80	48	IV
Egglestone et al,[8] 2020	21	68	24%	95%	5%	27	48	IV
Lachman et al,[17] 2018	29	58	45%	100%	0%	47	40	III
Wagener et al,[33] 2017	12	53	42%	100%	0%	94	83	IV
Kamrad et al,[34] 2015	73	55	60%	97%	3%	22	NA	III
Horisberger et al,[35] 2015	10	52	60%	100%	0%	72	48	IV
Roukis et al,[36] 2015	32	65	34%	94%	6%	77	26	IV
Hintermann et al,[37] 2013	117	55	48%	92%	8%	52	74	IV
Ellington et al,[38] 2013	41	60	71%	100%	0%	51	49	IV
Devries et al,[39] 2013	14	65	43%	100%	0%	94	29	IV
Median (Range)	26 (10–117)	59 (52–68)	44% (23%–71%)	99% (74%–100%)	1.5% (0%–26%)	72 (22–94)	48 (24–83)	IV (II–IV)

Implant Reoperation and Survival Rates

- The revision implants used in the 12 selected studies were
  - Hintegra: 141 (34%),
  - INBONE II: 80 (19%),
  - Agility: 64 (15%),
  - INBONE I: 45 (11%),
  - Others: 16 (4%), and not stated: 73 (17%).
- The median rate for
  - Infection was 4.8% (0%–19%) (11 studies),
  - Other procedures at the time of revision was 56.5% (0%–100%) (8 studies),
  - Reoperation was 16% (0%–41%) (12 studies), and
  - Conversion to fusion was 7% (0%–30%) (11 studies).
- Median implant survival was 86% (55%–100%) at a median follow-up of 4 (2–10) years (12 studies).
- The results are summarized in **Table 2**.

Clinical Outcomes

- Ten studies described the clinical outcome of revision TAA implants using the following PROMs: AOFAS,[13,17,33,35,37,38] VAS,[8,17,33,35,37,38] MOXFQ,[3,8,16,38] EQ5D,[3,34,38] FFI,[13,38] AOS,[8,38] SF-36,[17,34] and SMFA.[17] **Table 3** summaries the PROMs scores at follow-up in the selected studies.
- A significant postoperative improvement in the PROMs was recorded using the following scores: AOFAS in 4 studies,[17,33,35,37] VAS in 4 studies,[17,33,35,37] MOXFQ in 2 studies,[3,16] SF 36 in 1 study,[17] SMFA in 1 study,[17] and EQ5D in 1 study.[3]
- Four studies did not provide preoperative scores and it was not possible to examine the significance of the scores postoperatively.[8,13,34,38]
- Two studies did not provide any clinical outcomes in their articles.[36,39]

Radiographic Outcomes

The postoperative radiographic outcome of revision TAA is usually assessed by evaluating the implant for alignment of components, osteolysis, loosening, subsidence, and HO as described by Jamjoom and colleagues.[3] Almost all the selected studies had some deficient data relating to the radiographic outcomes at follow-up. Six studies did not provide any radiographic outcomes.[8,16,17,34,36,39] Of the 3 studies that reported the alignment of components results, only 1 reported a significant postoperative improvement in 3 out of 5 measures,[3] while 2 reported no change between the preoperative and postoperative assessments.[35,38] **Table 4** summarizes the reported radiographic outcomes at follow-up in the selected studies.

- The median (range) for osteolysis of
  - Tibia was 21% (6%–97%) and
  - Talus was 5%(0%–11%) (4 studies).[3,13,37,38]
- The median (range) for subsidence affecting
  - Tibia was 3% (2%–39%) and
  - Talus was 46% (28%–56%) (3 studies).[3,13,38]
- The median (range) for loosening affecting
  - Tibia was 7% (0%–38%) and
  - Talus was 21% (9%–44%) (3 studies).[3,13,37]
- The median (range) for HO was 21% (3%–33%) (4 studies).[2,33,35,37]

Table 2
Summary of the types of implants, complication, and survival rates in the selected studies

Author	Revision Implant Type (Number)	Infection Rate	Other Procedures Rate	Reoperation Rate	Conversion to Fusion Rate	Survival Rate
Jamjoom et al,[3] 2022	INBONE II (29)	7%	76%	0%	0%	97% at 3.3 y
Jennison et al,[16] 2021	INBONE II (15) Invision (3) Mix (5)	0%	9%	0%	0%	100% at 2 y
Behrens et al[13] 2020	INBONE I or II (18)	5.5%	72%	22.2%	6%	78% at 4 y
Egglestone et al,[8] 2020	INBONE (18) Hintegra (2) Infinity (1)	19%	NA	5%	5%	87% at 4 y
Lachman	INBONE I (5) INBONE II (18) Salto XT (3) Infinity (2) Star (1)	0%	NA	20.7%	6.9%	90% at 3.2 y
Wagener et al,[33] 2017	Hintegra (12)	8%	42%	8%	8%	92% at 6.9 y
Kamrad et al,[34] 2015	NA	NA	NA	41%	30%	76% at 5 y 55% at 10 y
Horisberger et al,[35] 2015	Hintegra (10)	0%	NA	33%	20%	80% at 4 y
Roukis et al,[36] 2015	Agility or Agility LP (23) INBONE II (8) Salto XT (1)	3%	56%	3%	NA	97% at 2 y
Hintermann et al,[37] 2013	Hintegra (117)	0.8%	57%	15%	6.8%	82% at 9 y
Ellington et al,[38] 2013	Agility (41)	4.8%	46%	17%	12%	82% at 4 y
Devries et al,[39] 2013	INBONE (14)	14.3%	100%	35.7%	7%	86% at 2.4 y

Table 3
Summary of patient reported clinical outcome scores at follow-up in the selected studies

Author, Year	Number of Revision TAA	PROMs	Summary of Findings
Jamjoom et al,[3] 2022	29	MOXFQ EQ5D	Post-op vs pre-op scores: significant improvement in 4 out of 4 domains (MOXFQ) and in 3 out of 6 domains (EQ5D)
Jennison et al,[16] 2021	23	MOXFQ	Post-op vs pre-op scores: significant improvement in 3 of 4 domains. Improvements in revision TAA was significantly less than primary
Behrens et al,[13] 2020	18	AOFAS FFI	No pre-op scores. Median post-op scores 74.5(AOFAS), 10.2 (FFI)
Egglestone et al,[8] 2020	21	MOXFQ AOS VAS	No pre-op scores. Median post-op scores 17 (MOXFQ), 12 (AOS), 10 (VAS). All scores were significantly better for revision TAA compared to arthrodesis
Lachman et al,[17] 2019	29	AOFAS, SF-36 SMFA, VAS	Post-op vs pre-op scores: significant improvement in all scores Primary TAA showed better improvement than revision (not significant).
Wagener et al,[33] 2017	12	AOFAS VAS	Post-op vs pre-op scores: significant improvement in median AOFAS VAS not recorded pre-op
Kamrad et al,[34] 2015	73	EQ5D SF-36	No pre-op scores. 15 out of 29 patients satisfied
Horisberger et al,[35] 2015	10	AOFAS VAS	Post-op vs pre-op scores: significant improvement in both scores
Hintermann et al,[37] 2013	117	AOFAS VAS	Post-op vs pre-op scores: significant improvement in both scores
Ellington et al,[38] 2013	41	MOXFQ, AOFAS, VAS AOS, FFI, EQ5D	No pre-op scores. No significant difference between revision TAA and conversion to fusion

Abbreviations: AOFAS, American Orthopaedic Foot and Ankle Society; AOS, ankle osteoarthritis scale; EQ5D, EuroQol-5 dimensions; FFI, foot function index; MOXFQ, Manchester-Oxford Foot Questionnaire; PROMs, patient-reported outcome measures; SF-36, short form 36; SMFA, short musculoskeletal function assessment; TAA, total ankle arthroplasty; VAS, visual analogue score.

Table 4
Summary of reported radiographic outcomes at follow-up in the selected studies

Author	Alignment	Osteolysis	Subsidence	Loosening	Heterotopic Ossification
Jamjoom et al,[3] 2022	Post-op to pre-op: significant improvement in 3/5 measures	Tibia 14% Talus 3%	Tibia 3% Talus. 28%	Tibia 0% Talus 21%	31%
Behrens et al[13] 2020	Post-op to pre-op: no significant improvement in 5 measures	Tibia 28% Talus 11%	Tibia 39% Talus 56%	Tibia 38% Talus 44%	NA
Wagener et al,[33] 2017	NA	0%	NA	0%	33%
Horisberger et al,[35] 2015	Stable, No formal measurements performed	NA	NA	NA	10%
Hintermann et al,[37] 2013	No comparison between pre-op and post-op	Tibia 6% Talus 6%	NA	Tibia 7% Talus 9%	3%
Ellington et al,[38] 2013	Post-op to pre-op: no significant improvement in 5 measures	Tibia 97% Talus 0%	Tibia 2% Talus 46%	NA	NA

DISCUSSION

With the increasing number of primary TAA implantations, failed TAA is becoming a regular challenge for foot and ankle surgeons. Nine of the 12 studies that reported outcomes of revision TAA in the literature so far were LOE-IV. These retrospective studies may not accurately reflect current techniques, technology, and outcomes, but they can still provide valuable information and serve as a benchmark for future improvements.

Indication for Revision

It is recognized that the indication for revision TAA can influence the outcome.[12,27] In a recent systematic review, Jennison and colleagues[12] showed that studies where revision TAA was performed for infection were associated with the highest risk of failure. Patients with periprosthetic infections often require a 2-stage procedure, are more likely to need soft tissue reconstructive procedures, and report lower PROMs scores at 2 years.[28] In this review, the 2 studies with the highest percentage of septic failed TAAs (Jennison and colleagues [26%][16] and Behrens and colleagues [11%][13]) either had a relatively short follow-up[16] or did not correlate the outcome with the indication for the revision.[13] Aseptic causes accounted for 95% (74%–100%) of the revision TAAs in the selected studies. The most common aseptic causes were loosening of 1 or 2 of the prosthetic components in 21% to 88%,[13,21] talar subsidence in 37.9% to 55.6%,[7,13] ankle deformity in 12% to 23.9%,[32,37] and progressive cyst formation in 15% to 17.6% of cases.[7,32]

Implant Utilized

The most used implants in revision TAA in the selected series were Hintegra (34%), INBONE I (11%), INBONE II (19%), and Agility (15%). INBONE II is the most utilized revision implant in studies published within the last 5 years. INBONE I and Agility are no longer available on the market. Hintegra is in its second generation which features a double hydroxyapatite coating and talar component pegs which resulted in a significant reduction in loosening rate from 26% to 5% in the reported data.[37] As a result of mixed heterogeneity of cases, the lack of detail, subgroup analysis, and standardized way for reporting complications and outcomes, at present the literature does not support any conclusions on the influence of the implant type on survival and complication rates.[12] **Fig. 1**A and B show the preoperative radiographs of a patient with a painful loose total ankle replacement. **Fig. 2**A and B show the postoperative radiographs of this patient following revision TAA using the INBONE II implant.

Complications

Several studies reported a higher complication rate for revision compared to primary TAA.[12,13,30] In a large database study by Lai and colleagues,[18] the incidence of wound complications following revision TAA was 19.7% compared to 9.3% after primary TAA. In a recent meta-analysis by Jennison and colleagues,[12] 14 papers were reviewed and showed that 26.9% of revision TAA required further surgical intervention. The authors found a median infection and reoperation rate of 4.8% and 16%, respectively.

Survival

Most results for revision TAA reports in the literature focused on short-term and medium-term outcomes. In our review of 12 studies, at a median follow-up of 4 years, the median reoperation and survival rates were 16% and 86%, respectively.

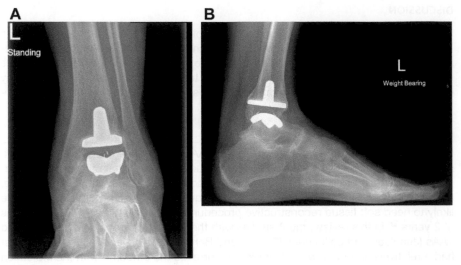

Fig. 1. (*A, B*) Preoperative radiographs of a patient with a painful loose total ankle replacement.

Hintermann and colleagues[37] has the largest series with the longest survival. The group reported a series of 117 revision TAAs and found cumulative survival at 5, 10, and 15 years are 81%, 74%, and 70%, respectively.[29,37] This was a single surgeon series at the design center and included 2 versions of the Hintegra implant.[37] The more recent reports with 2 to 3 year follow-up are showing promising results with survival at 90% to 100%.[3,16,17] It is therefore fair to say that in the current literature, there are several reports supporting the notion that in the short-term at least, the survival results of revision TAA could be considered comparable with primary procedures.[3,8,13,16]

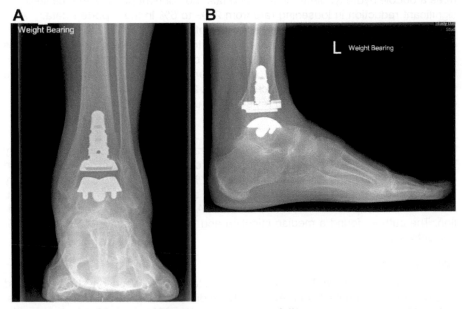

Fig. 2. (*A, B*) Postoperative radiographs of this patient following revision total ankle arthroplasty using the INBONE II implant.

Patient-Reported Outcome Measures

The authors observed that the 3 most frequently used PROMs in revision TAA series were AOFAS, VAS, and MOXFQ, although only 6 out of the 12 studies compared preoperative and postoperative scores. AOFAS is a scale that assesses pain, function, and range of motion in the ankle and hindfoot. It is the most commonly used and has been validated specifically for ankle arthroplasty.[25] MOXFQ is a validated 16-item outcome measure that analyses 3 domains (pain, walking/standing, and social interaction).[25] VAS is a simple scale used to measure pain intensity and has been widely used in patients who have undergone ankle replacement surgery.[25] In this review, significant postoperative improvements in the PROMs were recorded in all 3 measures,[3,16,17,33,35,37] The postoperative improvement in PROMs score following revision TAA was reported as better than arthrodesis for failed TAA[8] but did not rise to the levels seen with primary TAA.[17]

Radiographic Outcomes

Data relating to the radiographic outcomes of revision TAA are also very limited. Only 3 out of the 12 selected studies reported the alignment of components results,[3,35,38] with only 1 reporting a significant postoperative improvement in 3 out of 5 measures.[3]

Osteolysis, subsidence, and loosening were reported by a handful of studies and had a wide range.[3,13,37,38] It is worth noting that interpreting radiographs is highly subjective, and although criteria have been described by a number of authors, these measures can be difficult to quantify.[3,13,37] Therefore, the authors are unable to draw any real conclusions with the available data.

Limitations

There are numerous limitations to the study. There was extensive heterogeneity in the reporting of results and a considerable amount of data were missing. Most studies were small retrospective case series from a single center which implies potential selection and reporting bias. The follow-up was short in the majority of reports with only 3 studies reported a mean follow-up more than 5 years. There was wide range of implants used in the revision TAA by many surgeons in many centers creating a mixed group of study subjects. The PROMs tools used were wide-ranging, and the timing of performing the evaluation was not standardized. Radiographic outcomes were not adequately provided by most studies. Most studies did not provide relevant data such as range of movement.

SUMMARY

Revision TAA is a safe procedure that could produce good long-term patient outcome. At present, there are several reports supporting the notion that in the short-term, the results of revision TAA could be considered comparable with primary procedures. Nevertheless, data relating to long-term outcome are still limited in quantity and duration. Efforts should focus on preventing primary failure, with emphasis on ongoing surgeon training, patient selection, technique refinement, and technology advancement.

CLINICS CARE POINTS

- The majority of published outcomes of revision TAA were for an aseptic indication (95% of included patients).

- Revision TAA performed for a septic indication (infection) was associated with the highest risk of failure.
- INBONE I and II, Hintegra, and Agility were the most commonly used revision implants.
- The median infection and reoperation rates of revision TAA in our study were 4.8% and 16%, respectively.
- The median survival of revision TAA was 86% at a median 4 years.
- There are limited medium-term and long-term outcomes in the literature.
- The short-term implant survival results are comparable to primary TAA.
- PROMs in 6 of 12 studies improved from pre-revision to post-revision TAA, but the overall scores did not reach the level of primary TAA.
- Radiographic outcomes of revision TAA are limited and difficult to standardize.

REFERENCES

1. Kamrad I, Carlsson A, Henricson A, et al. Good outcome scores and high satidfaction rate after primary total ankle replacement. Acta Orthopaedica 2017;88(6):675–80.
2. Koivu H, Kohonen I, Mattila K, et al. Long term results of Scandinavian total ankle replacement. Foot Ankle Int 2017;38(7):723–31.
3. Jamjoom BA, Siddiqui BM, Salem H, et al. Clinical and Radiographic Outcomes of Revision Total Ankle Arthroplasty Using the INBONE II Prosthesis. J Bone Joint Surg Am 2022;104(17):1554–62.
4. Singh JA, Ramachandran R. Time trends in total ankle arthroplasty in the USA: a study of the National Inpatient Sample. Clin Rheumatol 2016;35(1):239–45.
5. NJR Reports Online source Available at https://reports.njrcentre.org.uk/ankles-all-procedures-activity. Accessed 15 January 2023.
6. Henricson A, Nilsson J-A, Carlsson A. 10-year survival of total ankle arthroplasties. Acta Orthopaedica 2011;82(6):655–9.
7. Brunner S, Barg A, Knupp M, et al. The Scandinavian total ankle replacement. J Bone Joint Surg Am 2013;95:711–8.
8. Egglestone A, Kakwani R, Aradhyula M, et al. Outcomes of revision surgery for failed total ankle replacement: revision arthroplasty versus arthrodesis. Int Orthopaedics 2020;44(12):2727–34.
9. Norvall DC, Ledoux WR, Shofer JB, et al. Effectiveness and safety of ankle arthrodesis versus arthroplasty. A prospective multicentre study. J Bone Joint Surg Am 2019;101:1485–94.
10. Ali AA, Forrester RA, O'Connor PO, et al. Revision of failed total ankle arthroplasty to a hindfoot fusion. Bone Joint J 2018;100-B:475–9.
11. Berkowitz MJ, Clare MP, Walling AK, et al. Salvage of failed total ankle arthroplasty with fusion using structural allograft and internal fixation. Foot Ankle Int 2011;32(5):493–502.
12. Jennison T, Spolton-Dean C, Rottenburg H, et al. The outcomes of revision surgery for a failed ankle arthroplasty : a systematic review and meta-analysis. Bone Jt Open 2022;3(7):596–606.
13. Behrens SB, Irwin TA, Bemenderfer TB, et al. Clinical and radiographic outcomes of revision total ankle arthroplasty using intramedullary referencing implant. Foot Ankle Int 2020;41(12):1510–8.

14. Henricson A, Carlsson A, Rydholm U. What is a revision of total ankle replacement? Foot Ankle Surg 2011;17(3):99–102.
15. Basques BA, Bitterman A, Campbell KJ, et al. Influence of surgeon volume on inpatient complication, cost, and length of stay following total ankle arthroplasty. Foot Ankle Int 2016;7(10):1046–51.
16. Jennison T, King A, Hutton C, et al. A Prospective Cohort Study Comparing Functional Outcomes of Primary and Revision Ankle Replacements. Foot Ankle Int 2021;42(10):1254–9.
17. Lachman JR, Ramos JA, Adams SB, et al. Patient-reported outcomes before and after primary and revision total ankle arthroplasty. Foot and ankle Internnational 2019;40(1):34–41.
18. Lai W, Arshi A, Ghorbanifarajzadeh A, et al. Incidence and predictors of early complications following primary and revision total ankle arthroplasty. Foot Ankle Surg 2019;25(6):785–9.
19. Cheung T, Din A, Zubairy A. Quality measure of total ankle replacement outcomes in a non-designer centre. J Orthopaedics 2020;20:286–92.
20. Escudero MI, Le V, Barahona M, et al. Total Ankle Arthroplasty Survival and Risk Factors for Failure. Foot Ankle Int 2019;40(9):997–1006.
21. Cody EA, Bejarano-Pineda L, Lachman JR, et al. Risk factors for failure of total ankle arthroplasty with minimum five years of follow up. Foot Ankle Int 2019; 40(3):249–58.
22. Gaugler M, Krähenbühl N, Barg A, et al. Effect of age on outcome and revision in total ankle arthroplasty. Bone Joint J 2020;102-B(7):925–32.
23. Hermus JP, Voesenek JA, van Gansewinkel EHE, et al. Complications following total ankle arthroplasty: A systematic literature review and meta-analysis. Foot Ankle Surg 2022;28(8):1183–93.
24. Onggo JR, Nambiar M, Phan K, et al. Outcome after total ankle arthroplasty with a minimum of five years follow-up: A systematic review and meta-analysis. Foot Ankle Surg 2020;26(5):556–63.
25. Shazadeh Safavi P, Janney C, Jupiter D, et al. A Systematic Review of the Outcome Evaluation Tools for the Foot and Ankle. Foot Ankle Spec 2019;12(5): 461–70.
26. Sansosti LE, Van JC, Meyr AJ. Effect of Obesity on Total Ankle Arthroplasty: A Systematic Review of Postoperative Complications Requiring Surgical Revision. J Foot Ankle Surg 2018;57(2):353–6.
27. Kunutsor SK, Barrett MC, Whitehouse MR, et al. Clinical Effectiveness of Treatment Strategies for Prosthetic Joint Infection Following Total Ankle Replacement: A Systematic Review and Meta-analysis. J Foot Ankle Surg 2020;59(2):367–72.
28. Conti MS, Irwin TA, Ford SE, et al. Patient-Reported Outcomes Following a Two-Stage Revision Total Ankle Arthroplasty for Chronic Periprosthetic Joint Infections. Foot Ankle Orthop 2022;7(4) 2473011421S00635.
29. Kvarda P, Susdorf R, Horn-Lang T, et al. Long-Term Survival of Hintegra Revision Ankle Arthroplasty in 116 Patients. Foot Ankle Orthop 2022;7(4). 2473011421S00737.
30. Nicolas AP, Ramaskandhan JR, Nurm T, et al. Outcomes of Revision Total Ankle Replacement: A Minimum of 2 Year Follow-up. Foot Ankle Orthop 2019;4(4). 2473011419S00320.
31. Schuberth JM, Christensen JC, Rialson JA. Metal-reinforced Cement augmentation for complex talar subsidence in failed total ankle arthroplasty. J Foot Ankle Surg 2011;50(6):766–72.

32. OCEBM Levels of Evidence. Oxford Centre for Evidence Based Medicine Available at: https://www.cebm.ox.ac.uk/resources/levels-of-evidence Accessed 15th January 2023.
33. Wagener J, Gross CE, Schweizer C, et al. Custom-made total ankle arthroplasty for the salvage of major talar bone loss. Bone Joint J 2017;99-B(2):231–6.
34. Kamrad I, Henricsson A, Karlsson MK, et al. Poor prosthesis survival and function after component exchange of total ankle prostheses. Acta Orthop 2015;86(4): 407–11.
35. Horisberger M, Henninger HB, Valderrabano V, et al. Bone augmentation for revision total ankle arthroplasty with large bone defects. Acta Orthop 2015;86(4): 412–4.
36. Roukis TS, Simonson DC. Incidence of Complications During Initial Experience with Revision of the Agility and Agility LP Total Ankle Replacement Systems: A Single Surgeon's Learning Curve Experience. Clin Podiatr Med Surg 2015; 32(4):569–93.
37. Hintermann B, Zwicky L, Knupp M, et al. HINTEGRA revision arthroplasty for failed total ankle prostheses. J Bone Joint Surg Am 2013;95(13):1166–74.
38. Ellington JK, Gupta S, Myerson MS. Management of failures of total ankle replacement with the agility total ankle arthroplasty. J Bone Joint Surg Am 2013;95(23):2112–8.
39. DeVries JG, Scott RT, Berlet GC, et al. Agility to INBONE: anterior and posterior approaches to the difficult revision total ankle replacement. Clin Podiatr Med Surg 2013;30(1):81–96.